A Straight Talking Introduction to

The Causes of Mental Health Problems

D1120523

First published 2010
Reprinted 2011

PCCS BOOKS Ltd
2 Cropper Row
Alton Road
Ross-on-Wye
Herefordshire
HR9 5LA
UK
Tel +44 (0)1989 763900
www.pccs-books.co.uk

**A Straight Talking Introduction to
the Causes of Mental Health Problems**

A CIP catalogue record for this book is available from the British Library

ISBN 978 1 906254 19 3

Cover designed in the UK by Old Dog Graphics
Typeset in the UK by The Old Dog's Missus
Printed in the UK by Ashford Colour Press, Gosport, Hampshire

Contents

Acknowledgements

John Read would like to acknowledge the many users of mental health services who have trusted him enough to share their understandings of the causes of their difficulties.

Pete Sanders owes a great debt to all of the patients and some of the staff he met in institutions in the late 1960s and early 70s. Their struggles to maintain and where possible celebrate human dignity in a plainly crazy system continue to help him make choices in life.

Introduction to the *Straight Talking* series

What are mental health problems?

Much of what is written and spoken about emotional distress or mental health problems implies that they are illnesses. This can lead us all too easily to believe that we no longer have to think about mental health problems, because illness is best left to doctors. They are the illness experts, and psychiatrists are the doctors who specialise in mental illness. This series of books is different because we don't think that all mental health problems should be automatically regarded as illnesses.

If mental health problems aren't necessarily illnesses, it means that the burden of responsibility for distress in our lives should not be entirely shouldered by doctors and psychiatrists. All citizens have a responsibility, however small, in creating a world where everyone has a decent opportunity to live a fulfilling life. This is a contentious idea, but one which we want to advance alongside the dominant medical view.

Rather than accept that solutions to mental health problems are 'owned' by the medical profession, we will take a good look at alternatives which involve the users of psychiatric services, their carers, families, friends and other 'ordinary people' taking control of their own lives. One of the tools required in order to become active in mental health issues, whether your own or other people's, is knowledge. This series of books is a starting point for anyone who wants to know more about mental health.

How these books are written

We want these books to be understandable, so we use everyday language wherever possible. The books could have been almost completely jargon-free, but we thought that including some technical and medical terms would be helpful. Most doctors, psychiatrists and psychologists use the medical model of mental illness and manuals to help them diagnose mental health problems. The medical model and the diagnostic manuals use a particular set of terms to describe what doctors think of as 'conditions'. Although these words aren't very good at describing individual people's experiences, they are used a lot in psychiatric and psychological services, so we thought it would be helpful to define these terms as we went along and use them in a way that might help readers understand what the professionals mean. We don't expect that psychiatrists and psychologists and others working in mental health services will stop using medical terminology (although we think it might be respectful for them to drop it when talking to their patients and their families), so these books should help you get used to, and learn *their* language.

The books also contain a few resources for further learning (pp. 157–8) as well as endnotes. These will not be important to everyone, but they do tell the reader where information – a claim about effectiveness, an argument for or against, or a quotation – has come from so you can follow it up if you wish.

Being realistic and reassuring

Our aim is to be realistic – neither overly optimistic nor pessimistic. Things are nearly always more complicated than we would like them to be. Honest evaluations of mental health problems, of what might cause them, of what can help, and of what the likely outcome might be, are, like so much in life, somewhere in between. For the vast majority of people it would be wrong to say that they have an illness from which they will never recover. But it would be equally wrong to say that they will be completely unchanged by the distressing thoughts and feelings they are having. Life is an accumulation of experiences. There is usually no pill, or any other treatment for that matter, that will take us back to 'how we were before'. There are many things we can do (and we will be looking at lots of them in this series) in collaboration with doctors, psychiatrists, psychologists, counsellors, indeed everyone working in mental health services, with the help of our friends and family, or on our own, which stand a good chance of helping us feel better and build a constructive life with hope for the future.

Of course, we understand that the experiences dealt with in these books can sometimes be so overwhelming, confusing and terrifying that people will try to escape from them by withdrawing, going mad or even by trying to kill themselves. This happens when our usual coping strategies fail us. We accept that killing oneself is, in some circumstances, a rational act – that for the person in question it can make a lot of sense. Nonetheless, we believe that much of the distress that underpins such an extreme course of action, from which there can be no turning back, is avoidable. For this reason, all of the books in this series point towards realistic hope and recovery.

Debates

There is no single convenient answer to many of the most important questions explored in these books. No matter how badly we might wish for a simple answer, what we have is a series of debates, or arguments more like, between stakeholders and there are many stakeholders whose voices demand space in these books. We use the word 'stakeholders' here because service users, carers, friends, family, doctors, psychologists, psychiatrists, nurses and other workers, scientists in drug companies, therapists, indeed all citizens, have a stake in how our society understands and deals with problems of mental health. It is simultaneously big business and intimately personal, and many things in between. As we go along, we try to explain how someone's stake in distress (including our own, where we can see it), whether business or personal, can influence their experience and judgement.

Whilst we want to present competing (sometimes opposing) viewpoints, we don't want to leave the reader high and dry to evaluate complicated debates on their own. We will try to present reasonable conclusions which might point in certain directions for personal action. Above all, though, we believe that knowledge is power and that the better informed you are, even though the information might be conflicting, the more able you will be to make sound decisions.

It's also useful to be reminded that the professionals involved in helping distressed people are themselves caught in the same flow of conflicting information. It is their *job*, however, to interpret it in our service, so that the best solutions are available to as many people as possible. You may have noticed that the word 'best' brings with it certain challenges, not least of all, what we mean when we use this term. Perhaps the best means the most effective? However, even using words like 'effective' doesn't completely clear up the puzzle. An effective treatment could be the one which returns someone to work quickly, if you are an employer, or one which makes someone feel happier and more calm, if they are your son or daughter. Readers will also know from recent press coverage that the National Institute for Health and Clinical Excellence (NICE) which evaluates and recommends treatments, keeps one eye on the budget, so 'effective' might mean 'cost effective' to some people. This brings us to evidence.

Evidence

Throughout these books there will be material which we will present as 'evidence'. This is one of the most contentious terms to be found in this series. One person's evidence is another person's fanciful mythology and yet another person's oppressive propaganda. Nevertheless the term crops up increasingly in everyday settings, most relevantly when we hear of 'evidence-based practice'. The idea behind this term is that the treatments psychologists and psychiatrists offer should be those that work. Crudely put, there should be some evidence that, say, talking about problems, or taking a prescribed drug, actually helps people to feel better. We encounter a real problem however, when trying to evaluate this evidence, as the books will demonstrate. We will try not to discount any 'evidence' out of hand, but we will evaluate it, and we will do this with a bias towards scientific evaluation.

    The types of evidence that will be covered in these books, along with their positive and negative points, include the following.

Research methods, numbers and statistics

On the one hand, the logic of most research is simple, but on the other hand, the way things have to be arranged to avoid bias in the results can lead to a perplexing system of measurements. Even the experts lose the sense of it sometimes. We'll try to explain the logic of studies, but almost certainly leave out the details. You can look these up yourself if you wish.

The books in this series look at research into a wide range of issues regarding mental health problems, including the experience of distress, what is known about the causes of problems, and their prevention and treatment. Different research methods are more or less appropriate for each of these areas, so we will be looking at different types of research as we go along. We say this now because many readers may be most familiar with studies into the *effective treatments* of distress, and we want to emphasise that there are many credible and valid sources of essential information about distress that are sometimes overlooked.

You may have come across the idea that some research methods are 'better' than others – that they constitute a 'gold standard'. In the case of research into the effectiveness of different treatments, the gold standard is usually considered to be 'randomised controlled trials' (RCTs). In simple terms, RCTs are complex (and often very expensive) experiments in which a group of individuals who all suffer from the same problem are randomly allocated to a treatment or a 'control' condition (at its simplest, no treatment at all) to see whether the treatment works. We are not necessarily convinced that RCTs always *are* the best way of conducting research into effective treatments, but they are, at the present time, the method given most credence by bodies which control funding, such as the National Health Service's National Institute of Health and Clinical Excellence (NICE), so we need to understand them.

Personal experience

Personal experience is an important source of evidence to the extent that nowadays, people who have suffered debilitating psychiatric distress are sometimes called 'experts by experience'.

Personal stories provide an essential counterbalance to the impersonal numbers and statistics often found in research projects such as RCTs. Whilst not everyone is average, by definition, most people are. Balancing the average results obtained from RCTs with some personal stories helps complete the picture and is now widely accepted to the extent that it has given birth to the new field of 'survivor research'.

Understanding contexts

Widening our view to include the families and lives of people, and the cultural, economic, social and political settings in which we live completes the picture. Mental health problems are connected to the conditions in which we all live, just as much as they are connected to our biology. From the start we want readers to know that, if there is one message or model which the books are trying to get across, it is that problems in mental health are more often than not the result of complex events in the environments in which we live and our reactions to them. These reactions can also be influenced by our biology or the way we have learned to think and feel. Hopefully these books will help disentangle the puzzle of distress and provide positive suggestions and hope for us all, whether we work in the system, currently have mental health problems ourselves, are caring for someone or are friends with someone who has.

We hope that readers of these books will feel empowered by what they learn, and thereby more able to get the best out of mental health services. It would be wonderful if our efforts, directly or indirectly, influence the development of services that effectively address the emotional, social and practical needs of people with mental health problems.

Richard Bentall
Pete Sanders
April 2009

Chapter 1
Our beliefs and values

Our thinking about the causes of mental health problems are, like our ideas about anything, shaped primarily by our life experiences. Although everything that follows in this book is supported by research findings (some of which we will describe as examples), different authors with different lives, and different beliefs and motives, could produce a very different book.

For example, John always starts his first lecture to a new student intake with a short personal history to show where his beliefs or, as some would say, 'biases', come from. This is his attempt to demonstrate that despite all the research studies that we will be covering later, everyone's beliefs about what causes human distress, madness and so on are really still just beliefs. And those beliefs come largely from our life experiences, from the beliefs of other people whom we trust and respect and various other 'subjective' rather than 'objective' sources. Our backgrounds go some way to explain our beliefs about the causes of mental health problems.

John writes:
Looking back, I now realise that one of the reasons I went into mental health work was that it was reassuring to know there were people more screwed up than myself. At the time, however, I simply thought I wanted to help people. I guess I also preferred the helper role to the helpee role.

Safer? Perhaps because I was part-way bonkers myself, or could at least understand why one might want to kill oneself, I seemed to be quite good at connecting to people in extreme states of distress, despair and confusion. I was more fascinated than scared (but sometimes only just) when people heard voices I couldn't hear, or had weird beliefs about people being out to get them. I was sufficiently paranoid myself in those years that when the psychiatrist in the New York hospital where I was working complimented me on my ability to build relationships with even the most 'psychotic' people, and asked me how I did it, I was so convinced that he was taking the piss that I slithered away to cry in the staff room. A kind nurse used her own considerable skills to convince me I had been wrong and that she too thought I was pretty good at the job.

Anyway here are just three of the stories about how I came to believe that 'bad things happening' is usually sufficient explanation for 'mental health problems' and why asking the person concerned what they think is going on can be better than thinking you've explained something by throwing a diagnostic label, or a biological theory, at it.

He had been on the ward for three days without opening his eyes. No mean feat. The doctors had been trying to figure this out, but 'eye-closed behaviour' just wasn't anywhere to be found in the diagnostic manual. One night, about 2 a.m., I asked him, more from boredom than clinical judgement, why he kept his eyes shut. He immediately opened them, put his face uncomfortably close to mine, and said 'It's about fucking time one of you idiots asked me that!' He then explained to me that he had been put in the hospital, against his will, to get 'insight' and that's what he had been doing!

Just before my very first chance to help run the weekly group therapy session, an old woman approached me to explain that she wouldn't be talking in the group because she thought that whatever she had said in the past in the group had always been turned into a 'symptom' and used against her. She explained that she didn't want me to be offended by her silence. (I think she could see I was nervous.) After the group I retreated to the staff team where the patients' performance in the group was evaluated. There, the woman's not speaking was interpreted by the rest of the team as a sure sign of her paranoia.

I was 'specialing' a teenage girl. This meant being locked in with her in the 'quiet room' (the noisiest place on the ward) to make sure she didn't try, again, to kill herself by smashing her head into the wall. She hadn't spoken for weeks. A 'catatonic schizophrenic'. Having had no training I tried: 'It's OK if you don't want to talk, but if you do that's OK too.' She didn't. She said nothing for the whole two hours. The next day we were locked in again. This time she started to speak but stopped after just one word: 'My ....' The next day she said 'father'. OK, I thought, I can do this – one word a day. The next day, however, she reverted to silence for the two hours. The next day she said 'me'. Now we had 'My father … me.' The missing word, I learned later from a family meeting, was 'raped'.

It all seemed rather simple to me. The people in the hospital had had bad, sometimes horrific, experiences and were reacting to them in perfectly understandable ways. But they are only understandable if you know what has happened. And they will only tell you what has happened if you are genuinely interested and show that you will listen. If, on the other hand, you start from the premise that they have some terrible illness or are irreversibly mad and that what they say is just a symptom of that illness, disorder or madness, then you can't easily establish the relationship necessary to be told what has happened. This becomes a self-fulfilling prophecy. Without knowing what has gone on in a person's life, and how they have made sense of it for themselves, some people's ways of coping with it all can indeed look a bit strange, even totally crazy.

The diagnoses that the psychiatrists and psychologists spent so much time deciding on, and the theories about genetics and brain dysfunction that always seemed to accompany them, never made much sense to me. They always, from that first job in New York, seemed to create the illusion of an explanation while explaining nothing at all. I remember asking a psychiatrist how he knew that a woman we were discussing had 'schizophrenia'. 'Because she has the symptoms of schizophrenia,' he replied. 'How do you know they are the symptoms of schizophrenia?' I continued. The psychiatrist answered, 'Because they are the things that schizophrenics do.' The explanation was accompanied by such an air of certainty that there seemed no point continuing the conversation. I liked this particular psychiatrist very much. He was caring and intelligent, and very supportive of this naïve 22-year-old despite all my silly questions. But there seemed, to me, to be a major flaw in this circular thinking.

As I progressed on through my training as a clinical psychologist and numerous jobs as a psychologist and as a manager of mental health services, my beliefs about the causes of human distress have been repeatedly reinforced. They have been further reinforced since re-entering academia in 1994 by my studies and my own research.

4

Of course, it is quite possible that I am guilty of precisely what I often accuse overly biological psychiatrists of doing. Perhaps, like Simon and Garfunkel, I just 'see what I want to see and disregard the rest'. Certainly for years I was vehemently 'opposed' to any theories about brains and genes – having seen the damage done to people's lives by these theories' minimising, or ignoring altogether, the social causes of distress and despair. So I try to be honest about my biases. I think that is better than pretending that in the difficult task of answering the question 'what causes mental health problems?' it is possible to be completely scientific and 'objective'.

———

Pete writes:

In my mid-to-late teens I got successive holiday jobs in both a local psychiatric hospital and (as it was known then) a 'hospital for the mentally subnormal'. As a 17-year-old from a family with no real exposure to mental health problems, my first day was like a descent into hell. I was overwhelmed by the sights, sounds and smells of the place. I had no way of understanding any of it – it was profoundly disturbing. Nevertheless, I knuckled down and go on with the job – to be a 'nursing assistant'. I did everything from helping patients with everyday care such as feeding, shaving, washing and going to the toilet through to sitting on someone whilst they were injected with paraldehyde. I am still haunted by the smell.

When I was 18, my father died suddenly of a heart attack, three weeks before my A-level exams. He was just 48 years old. I was a pretty happy-go-lucky lad until this happened – it was my first experience of real loss in my life. The family (my 14-year-old brother, my Mom and me) were close and my Dad had always been a very 'hands-on' father.

Shocking and completely unexpected, Dad's death completely knocked the stuffing out of me. I really didn't know how to carry on, and our wider family (uncles, aunts, grandmothers, etc.) were also profoundly affected because Dad was the youngest of five. On the day of the funeral, just after the service at the crematorium, my uncle took me to one side and told me that I was the man of the family now. He told me that in order to make my Dad proud I must look after my Mom and brother, pass my A-levels and go to university. It seemed quite reasonable at the time. I reckoned I was doing quite well really.

My dad died a minute or two after midnight. At the hospital Mom and I were ushered into a waiting room and shortly a pleasant nurse came in and said, 'I'm sorry, we've lost him Mrs Sanders' whilst she quickly pressed a tablet into my hand (I was sobbing by then) and said, 'This will help'. It was Librium (chlordiazepoxide, a benzodiazepine tranquilliser).

From then I was on autopilot, chemically insulated from grief, and did exactly what my uncle said I must. I still can't remember the next three weeks, nor the exams, nor the rest of the summer, and it wasn't till I got to university to study psychology and sought some solace in drugs that I hit the ground hard. I later realised that I had suffered a psychotic episode. The GP at the university health centre was an incredibly kind man who clearly thought he had a talent for psychiatry and I later learned he was renowned for not referring people to specialist services if he thought he didn't really have to. In my case, this was a godsend. He listened to me ramble (sometimes very late into the night), prescribed some antipsychotic meds but stopped them pretty soon when he thought I was doing OK. He helped me manage my own experiences (sometimes not too well, and sometimes I needed help) and it was his encouragement to take control of my life that restored me to a reasonable balance. Some people might think that he was the father to me that I was missing so much. Who knows? In my ramblings with him, I began to put some pieces together about my buried experiences of grief and loss, but it took time – most of the rest of my time as an undergraduate.

As I wrestled with terrible anxiety and very frightening strange thoughts, I remembered my time as a nursing assistant and realised that another GP might have had me committed to a mental hospital. I believed I had had a very lucky escape. All of this made me an avid consumer of literature on psychology and psychiatry. And, as I learned more, in the early 70s I went to antipsychiatry meetings and decided that I wanted to help other people in the way the university health centre doctor helped me. I thought, based on my own experience, that people should be helped to self-manage and understand their experiences, not have them chemically suppressed. It might take time, but, with luck and kindness it leads to a lasting healing.

Our beliefs and values

So one of your tasks, as a reader of this book, is to remember that your authors come to the issues with a set of clearly formed opinions. We suspect, however, that you do too. The difference is that you are open-minded enough to be reading the book, in hope of some new ideas, rather than writing it in hope of sharing ideas that have been held by the authors for decades.

Regardless of what you may want to believe about the relative importance of personal histories and scientific evidence, the research literature about the causes of mental health problems is a bit like the Bible in two ways.

Firstly, most of it is disputed – whatever it says – mostly because science progresses through trying to prove hypotheses wrong and the ensuing debate is expected to take us closer to the truth. This makes life very interesting if you are a scientist, but not so great if you or someone close to you is suffering mental distress and you want answers you can trust, answers that will last (not be superseded next year by new evidence), in short, answers that will help.

Secondly, the range of evidence is so broad and diverse, and in places downright contradictory, that you can almost always find stuff to support your own beliefs. We think that mental health researchers who believe they are immune to this sort of bias – i.e., who believe that they are purely objective scientists – are kidding themselves. Naturally if you have suffered distress, or have cared for a friend or relative who has suffered, these experiences will shape your beliefs. And just as surely, those of us whose job involves caring for people who are suffering distress will have both personal beliefs and professional beliefs (we like to call them 'theories').

If we look back at our lives we can develop all sorts of theories about what caused us to be the way we were as children, teenagers and adults. Especially if we have suffered any kind of hardship, bullying, emotional, physical and/or sexual abuse or other trauma. We guess every one of you reading this could come up with a list of childhood, teenage and adult events that you think had an effect on the sort of person you were then, and are today. All of these experiences will contribute to your understanding of distress, madness, mental illness, and will even determine what terms you use to describe it.

Ways of thinking about causes

This book is about possible causes of what are often called 'mental illnesses'. This sentence takes us straight away to an important issue. Our thinking about the different mental experiences of people as *illnesses* is only one of many possible ways of understanding what might be happening. Yet it is a way that is so natural to many of us that most of us think it is a fact about the world. We are inviting the readers of this book to try to step back from these assumptions about what is true and take a new look. Why? In the first place, human experiences are extremely variable and complex. This points to the causes being equally complex, however comforting and convenient it would be if the causes were more simple. Starting out thinking that different experiences are illnesses will artificially narrow our search. We would tend to simply get what we set out to find, rather than find what might actually be there.

Secondly, we have to accept that our understanding of just about everything in the world, however expert we are in a subject, is an unfinished work in progress. Current explanations of mental experiences are the best guesses we have at the present. We realise this could be upsetting if readers are looking for reassurance in the face of overwhelming upset, fear and chaotic thinking.

Thirdly, it gives us all an opportunity to discover something new about human beings. We think it's best to be honest from the outset and say that we, along with every other mental health professional, are still learning about human psychology. There are very few things that even the best experts are sure about. In a very real sense this is upsetting to many of us. Whenever we are frightened or upset, it is perfectly natural to seek reassurance and probably the first thing we look for are the answers to the questions 'What is happening?' and 'Why is this happening?' What this book offers, in the face of uncertainty, is a way of thinking that is positive, hopeful and critical. We hope it is helpful too.

The nature of psychological distress

Feeling distressed and being different

It is often said that everyone is different. Yet being *too* different makes a person stick out in the crowd and this can be uncomfortable, to say the least. Being seen as 'different' is often the catalyst for bullying at school, attracts unwelcome attention as an adult and, depending upon the 'difference', can even lead to a diagnosis of mental illness.

Taking sexuality as an example, until 1973, being gay was a diagnosable mental illness in the *Diagnostic and Statistical Manual of Mental Disorders*, third edition (DSM-III) published by the American Psychiatric Association (APA). Now that psychiatry has caught up with society, it is clear to us all that different sexualities are just that, *differences* between people, not an indication of *illness*. Differences in sexuality are expressions of human individuality that should be celebrated, not diagnosed. When people are judged as bad or ill simply because they are different, the resulting stigmatisation can, in turn, make a person feel so distressed, ashamed and isolated that they experience symptoms that could be diagnosed as, e.g., 'depression'.

Studies show that a higher than usual number of, for example, gay men attempt suicide.[1,2] This is a terrible double whammy which directly results from natural differences being judged negatively, then, instead of explaining that such differences are simply expressions of human variation, we find that medicine and psychiatry make things worse by telling us these experiences are illnesses; that there is something sick or defective about us.

It's also true that even people's experiences of being different are, well, different. That is to say that most people will be comfortable with being different in some respects, but not others. Everyone has different tolerance levels but for most of us it is particularly difficult to endure being different in a way that attracts unwelcome attention in the form of bullying, discrimination and other forms of stigmatisation. It is not 'character building'. So if significant professional groups in society, the media and psychiatric diagnosis manuals say that being gay is an unacceptable difference, it's likely that the experience of being gay will be deeply unpleasant for many people simply because of the bullying, discrimination and stigmatisation that it attracts. Take away that unpleasant discrimination and differences in sexuality have a much better chance of being experienced with joy. We'll look at how stigmatisation and discrimination affect our happiness and mental health in Chapters 5 and 6.

Who is upset by distressing experiences?

Another problem with psychological distress is that it is sometimes as upsetting to witness it or have to deal with someone who is panicking, chaotic, agitated or overwhelmed, as it is to be suffering from any or all of these things. Someone behaving in a strange or disturbed way can be disturbing to those around them. Many, but not all, people who suffer extremely upsetting experiences are painfully aware that their behaviour has a disturbing effect on those around them, causing them further distress. As a result they might keep themselves to themselves more, and this social isolation (a reasonable response to the world) is itself often seen as a diagnosable symptom of 'illness'.

If you are a witness to disturbing behaviour you will most likely feel differently depending upon whether the person in question is:

- a close friend or relative
- a life partner or spouse
- a passing member of the public
- the same or different ethnicity as you
- a man or a woman
- a child, adolescent or adult

Each person has their own emotional reaction to disturbing behaviour and tries to make some rational sense of it according to their personal and professional perspective – some of us will have a professional role, such as psychiatric nurse, social worker or police officer. Each response will, in some part, be determined by our beliefs about what causes psychological disturbance in general, and what has caused this distressing episode in particular. And each response will have the potential to help the distressed person or make them feel worse.

A key question is 'How distressed is the person whose behaviour is so disturbing to me?' Not everyone who is disturbed is disturbing and not everyone who is disturbing is disturbed. It's not sensible to think that everyone behaving in a disturbing way should be diagnosed with a mental illness. What we experience as disturbing from moment to moment, situation to situation, is determined by many factors, including what we think is normal and the strength of our desire to live a quiet life, free from threat.

All these complexities are conveniently brushed under the carpet by the illness model which has it that behaviour X is a symptom of illness Y. From this perspective, if you want to understand what is going on the answer seems seductively simple: Y is causing X. This is not only far *too* simple, it can be dangerous. There is also a tendency in many societies to use the term 'mental illness' to identify and deal with people, behaviour and even ideas which are disturbing to the rest of us. We have already looked very briefly at how society included psychiatric diagnoses as a way of dealing with people who disturbed the comfortable norm in the case of sexuality. In their book *Making Us Crazy*, Kutchins and Kirk[3] describe how the diagnosis 'masochistic personality disorder' was very nearly included in the DSM-III-R.[4] Masochistic Personality Disorder was purported (by a panel of psychiatrists) to be the tendency of people (mainly women) to provoke violence against them. So a woman complaining of domestic violence could have been diagnosed with a supposed condition in which she somehow *invited* violence towards her.

We will see throughout the book how ideas about what causes 'mental illness' are, at least in part, defined by the prevailing cultural beliefs in any particular society.

Psychological distress and illness

Western science and most folk in the developed world take the general view that mind and body are separate, which comes from a very long tradition of philosophy called dualism. Our present-day ideas were set out by French philosopher René Descartes in the 17th century. Believing that mind and body are separate lays the foundation of the idea that our minds are unaffected by events in our bodies and vice versa. But we know from a mountain of scientific and personal evidence that when something happens in our body, it can affect the way we think and feel (both positively and negatively, and to different degrees). We also know that some experiences affect the way our body works, such as anxiety (e.g., racing heart, feeling light-headed, breathless, tunnel vision). These links between mind and body then form chains – for example, being involved in a traumatic event will cause anxiety. Anxiety brings about very strong physical responses which themselves can be disturbing. This leads to more anxiety. If this spiral of anxiety continues over a period of time we might call it 'stress' which in turn affects the amount of a hormone, cortisol, which in turn, if released over a long period will weaken the immune system. And so on … This is one (highly simplified) example of the many interactions and overlappings between mind and body which are a necessary part of life, but can sometimes cause problems.

In short, we don't understand how our body and what we know as 'mind' actually bring about our experiences. This makes it genuinely difficult to separate the physical from the psychological and this difficulty is important when we try to work out whether the physical and psychological events we find distressing are actually 'illnesses'.

When we feel overwhelmed by distressing feelings and chaotic thoughts we can easily think we are suffering from an illness with a physical dimension. There can be real benefits in understanding experiences in this way:

- it gives access to a shared vocabulary – lots of people speak the language of mental *illness* (not only doctors and other experts, but also probably friends and relatives)
- it helps a person to fit in – they will not feel so isolated
- it gets access to funding for treatments (both physical, i.e., medications, and psychological talking treatments)

However, many people, professionals and members of the public, do not think of these unpleasant experiences as an indication of *illness* at all, let alone in a similar way to a physical illness. Some think that such experiences don't indicate that there is anything at all wrong with the person having them – they think of the experiences as being simply different. Possibly unusual and probably upsetting, but nevertheless only another expression of the range of human experience. The Mad Pride[5] movement promotes the idea that to have different experiences is simply an expression of diversity, and that the person having these experiences is made to feel ill by the stigmatising way society and other people respond.

In this book we invite you to consider how logical it is to think of distressing experiences as illnesses, rather than reasonable responses to an unreasonable environment. When we say 'reasonable' response, we don't mean that all reasonable responses are necessarily immediately understandable to everyone. We think that the experiences and behaviour of people in distress are always meaningful to the person having them. We also think that understanding your own experiences better, and someone else understanding you too, is often the first step to feeling better. Finally, we challenge the evidence that they are caused by biological factors or chemical imbalances of the sort suggested in the majority of textbooks and in the media. You can make your mind up for yourself.

Our own experience as the basis of explanations

Many readers will know someone who has had a 'nervous breakdown' or suffers from a 'mental illness'. Many of you will have had experiences yourselves which have been diagnosed as depression, anxiety, schizophrenia etc. Others will have only come across the ideas in conversation, or in the media. We have already suggested that your personal history will affect your ideas, and accepting that, we would like you to try to answer the following questions, based on your own experience. Is extreme human distress caused by:

- people being born with a faulty brain or nervous system?

- people being too sensitive and needing to toughen up emotionally in order to deal with today's world?

- a form of demonic possession?

- people being born with a tendency to respond in certain ways to stress, which will show itself if they have certain experiences, like bereavement, separation and divorce, or childbirth?

- people growing up in chaotic, crazy families?

- people learning unhealthy ways of dealing with events in their lives which lead to upsetting symptoms when distressing events happen to them?

- a lack of spiritual strength or lack of disciplined faith?

- child abuse or traumatic events in childhood?

We will look later at the evidence for many of these possible understandings. Some we can explain by looking at the history of ideas about the world and see that some understandings of madness are inextricably bound up with the zeitgeist or 'spirit of the times'. It could be that some common understandings of madness turn out to be as realistic as believing that the earth is flat. In Chapter 2, therefore, we try to place ideas in history. Whatever else history can teach us, we must learn to understand our own biases in the way we look at the world and see if that interferes with our ability to understand other people's experiences.

What you won't find in this book

Although this book is about the causes of mental health problems, we think that some readers will quite naturally want to link causes to treatments. If we know what causes distress, the next logical step is to turn our knowledge about causes into devising treatments to help people feel better. We have tried, however, to stick to our task and readers will not find much about treatments in this book. For an honest evaluation of psychological treatments for mental health problems, we suggest readers take a look at David Pilgrim's book with that title in this series.[6] We are also sure that people will devise their own theories about what may or may not help their friend, relative or themselves, based on their own exploration of possible causes.

Another thing you will not find in this book is a catalogue of categories of 'disorder', or lists of symptoms, with a further list of possible causes for each one. We don't have the space to include a comprehensive review of possible causes of each symptom or diagnostic category that might be found in the DSM-IV-TR[7] for example. We realise that this, too, might be frustrating for readers who want answers quickly because either they or their friends or family are in extreme distress. There are two further reasons why we have not done this. Firstly, it would almost certainly not be useful because, as we have hinted already, each part of the list would be filled with unresolvable debates. Secondly, we think that given the current disputes and debates, the best way of understanding an individual person's mental health problem is to understand that person. All aspects of their life, past and present are likely to hold clues as to why they are thinking and feeling the way they do. Nothing is automatically ruled out, and just as importantly, nothing is automatically ruled in.

We think this way of trying to understand mental health problems stands the best chance of locating real causal factors for each person. Furthermore it lets us acknowledge that causal factors might well not be single events (a biological malfunction, or experience of abuse) but might be sequences or accumulations of events.

Chapter 2
A brief history of beliefs about the causes of human distress

Thinking about the history of how people have, in the past, thought about the causes of human distress, despair, madness and so on can be surprisingly helpful when trying to understand our own problems today. Others have done this in more detail.[1,2,3]

Firstly, history reminds us that there are many different ways to think about the causes. This can help us avoid getting stuck on just one, perhaps simplistic, explanation. Secondly, we can see that, although we do have more scientific approaches today than in the past, a big factor in determining which type of explanation dominates at any particular time and place is the world-view operating in that time and place. Furthermore, we can see that the dominant idea about how distress is caused can be useful to those with political or economic power. The flip side of that is that the theories (and the treatments justified by the theories) are often targeted at relatively powerless groups, such as women and poor people. People who simply don't fit in, who break 'social norms', can be described as mad and causal theories are developed by 'experts' to prove that, and to explain why they need 'treatments' to be made more normal.

Lastly, we learn that there are three general types of causal theory that have been battling away with one another for centuries. These three are nature, nurture and religion. The nature position argues either that people are born with problems or that the problems are caused by some malfunctioning in the body (often, but not always, the brain). The nurture, or environmental, position claims that we develop problems because of the bad things that happen to us, or by the absence of good things that should have happened but didn't. The religious position can involve punishment by the gods, but also sometimes involves the notion of people just being bad or immoral. Another dimension along which causal theories vary is whether to hold the individual responsible for their own problems.

Gods and devils

Four thousand years ago 'madness' was thought to result from the evil influence of some enemy, real or imagined. The world-view in Mesopotamia around 2,000 BC included the belief that evil demons were responsible for ailments and the source of recovery was the appropriate good god. It was the demon responsible for madness. She was assisted by a collection of lesser demons and sorcerers and the whole department was answerable to Ishtar, the female god supervising all witchcraft and evil.[4] The Persians and Hindus also held evil gods – Ahriman and Siva – accountable for strange behaviours.

The earliest recorded attempts of the Hebrews to understand insanity also reflected the prevailing world-view.[5,6] Moses was clear about one cause: 'The Lord will smite thee with madness'.[7] Moses also came close to providing an early example of this book's central theme – that madness is caused primarily by adverse life experiences: 'You shall be only oppressed and crushed continually; so that you shall be driven mad by the sight which your eyes shall see.'[8] The ancient Hebrew theory remains, however, one of divine punishment since it is the Lord, rather than life events, that did the oppressing and crushing.

The world-view of the ancient Hebrews, in the Old Testament, included the notion that an efficient way to eradicate abnormal behaviour was to eliminate the person rather than just the behaviour. 'A man or woman who is a medium or a wizard shall be put to death; they shall be stoned with stones, their blood shall be upon them.'[9] The reason given by Moses for punishing a long list of behaviours by death was: 'So you shall purge the evil from Israel.'[10] Whether 'Israel' refers to a race or a country, this represents an early version of the primitive tendency to cleanse or eliminate unacceptable differences. Sometimes in history it has been 'graced' by the genetic theory of unacceptable behaviour and the eugenic approach to eradicating madness via the creation of a genetically untainted race.[11]

By the time of the first drafts of the Talmud (70–200 AD), the Hebrew world-view had changed. Now, before anyone can be punished for their behaviour, they must be considered responsible for it. While the Old Testament clearly held madness to be the direct result of sinning, the Talmud argues that the 'mad' are 'not responsible for the damage or the shame they produce'. They must, therefore, be helped rather than stoned or purged.[12,13]

The introduction of reason

Thinkers in Greece had also indulged in magical and religious theories about unusual behaviour. Whether it was Ajax killing a flock of sheep believing it to be the enemy, or the daughters of Proteus believing they were cows and acting accordingly, there was a god to blame.[14]

There followed in Greece, however, what many describe as the most significant change in world-view that humanity has experienced. The 'Classical Era' was marked by the replacement of supernatural explanations with observation and reason. Priests were gradually replaced by physicians. The most famous doctor of all time, Hippocrates (460–377 BC), was among the first to promote the 'medical model' of madness. He produced the first of its many attempts to reduce the complexities of unusual, distressed or distressing human behaviours to a set of categories of illness each with its own physiological cause:

> Men ought to know that from the brain and from the brain only arise our pleasures, joys, laughters and jests. ... Those who are mad through phlegm are quiet, and neither shout nor make a disturbance; those maddened through bile are noisy, evil-doers, and restless, always doing something inopportune.[15]

Hippocrates was just as convinced then as biological psychiatry is today that he really was discovering the physical causes of illnesses, rather than promoting a simplistic theory that conceals the complexities, and justifies and camouflages the social control of, unacceptable or disturbing behaviour. A sect called the Dogmatists was certainly convinced. It was dedicated to prohibiting any investigation beyond the biological ideology of the day, because they argued that Hippocrates had already discovered everything worth discovering. This attitude of certainty has been a feature of human thinking throughout history and remains so today in many areas of life. Any 'dogmatic' belief in a single system of explanation to the exclusion of any evidence to the contrary stymies discussion and sometimes even renders reasonable debate impossible. Whilst the current book definitely *leans* toward psychological and social explanations of causes, we do not wish to prevent debate by proposing a fundamentalist psychosocial theory. Quite the contrary.

The *World History of Psychiatry*[16] offers an insight, still valuable today, into one motivation for simplistic biological theories. The Greeks were becoming aware of human conflicts; not only internal conflicts regarding the motivations underpinning human behaviour such as the 'reasoning' versus 'desiring' conflict identified by Plato (427–347 BC) over 2000 years before Freud, but also the conflict between the individual and the demands of society (see discussion of the 'id' versus the 'superego' in Chapter 7). In the absence of religious instructions regarding such dilemmas there was a need to identify other forces over which the individual had little control and for which they could not be held accountable:

> The Hippocratic model of mental illness and of its treatment may have provided an important source of relief of anxiety, guilt and responsibility, by translating inner conflicts and dissonances into physiological and physicalistic terms.[17]

Hippocrates' treatments probably were effective in altering behaviour. We both think we might have been less quiet or noisy, and would have agreed that our behaviour was biologically based, rather than face being forced to vomit or defecate uncontrollably, or to swallow hellebore – a poison now used in insecticides – especially if we knew that, if all that failed, blood-letting was the treatment of last resort.

During this period there was a fading of an extreme male dominance that had included, for example, the feeding of boys at the expense of girls. When Plato wrote 'within the woman there is a wild, animalistic, Bicchantic [sic], frenzied creature, who must be gratified, or else she goes beserk',[18] he wasn't suggesting that generations of oppression had led to pent-up anger, nor that such oppression can drive women mad. He was laying the foundations of a quite different type of theory of female madness, a theory in keeping with the physiological explanations of the time, one that could be used not to liberate women but to continue their oppression.

The invention of 'hysteria' is an early example of the repeated, and continuing, use of biological theories of madness to force women into the roles determined for them by men.

> Whenever the womb – which is an indwelling creature desirous of child-bearing – remains without fruits long beyond the due season, it is vexed and takes it ill; and by straying all ways through the body and blocking up the passages of the breath and preventing the respiration it casts the body into the uttermost distress, and causes, moreover, all kinds of maladies until the desires and love of the two sexes unite them.[19]

The treatments of choice for 'hysteria' were marriage and fumigation of the vagina. Although the experts told their 'patients' that the purpose of the 'treatment' was to attract the wandering uterus back to its rightful place, we can see with hindsight that it was the wandering of women from their subservient role that was the real concern.

A return to religion

The social structure of the mighty Roman Empire eventually crumbled before an onslaught of epidemics and marauding barbaric tribes. The resulting insecurity led to a return to supernatural beliefs. By the 4th century AD, Emperor Constantine had made Christianity the official religion. The Church and State become an inseparable and immense power. In the field of madness, observation, reason and physiological theories were replaced with variations of the old religious themes. The Church became protector of the infirm and insane.

In the search for some external, and preferably heavenly, force to explain madness, it was thought that people tended to be particularly weird when alone at night, thus obviously, the moon was responsible for craziness. Mad people have, ever since, been called 'lunatics'.

Another concept, more consistent with Christianity, explained almost any anxiety-provoking event, including epidemics, conflagrations and madness. It was called witchcraft and it offers one of the most horrifying examples of the violence that can be justified by theories about groups of people considered defective. The target group is typically that which best symbolises the nature of a society's collective anxiety.

The extent to which cultural changes affect theories about whom or what is to blame for madness is well illustrated if we divide the Middle Ages (roughly the 5th – 15th century) into two periods. In the earlier period causal theories were influenced by the charitable aspects of Christianity. Care was relatively humane. Patients of the original Bethlehem Hospital in London (also variously known as St. Mary Bethlehem, Bethlem Hospital, Bethlehem Hospital and later to degenerate into the Bedlam 'snake-pit') wore arm badges when granted a pass out of the hospital. The response was so positive that people often counterfeited badges for themselves so that other people thought they were inmates. During this period people accused of being possessed by the devil were not held personally responsible. The treatment of choice, exorcism, was not, therefore, a punitive process aimed at the individual, but a benevolent one directed against the real cause of the problem – the Devil.

However, from the 11th century onwards the breakdown of feudal structures, accompanied by insurrections, often aimed at the Church, demanded a set of scapegoats. Public trials and executions might deter other potential 'heretics', but possessed women could not serve this purpose if they were not responsible for their actions. By the time Kraemer and Sprenger published their witch-hunting manual, *Malleus Maleficarum* (1486), it was 'discovered' that witches voluntarily invite the Devil into their lives. Now that people were deemed personally responsible, the treatment of choice was to annihilate the host.

Religious and social factors during this latter period of the Middle Ages had created an intense fear and hatred of women and a fiercely misogynist Church. The *Malleus Maleficarum* described women as 'a foe to friendship, an unescapable punishment, a necessary evil, a natural temptation, a desirable calamity … an evil of nature painted with fair colours.'[20] Consequently, the vast majority of people tortured and murdered were, indeed, women.[21] Many of them were guilty of nothing more than being sought after for their healing skills. Their herbs and brews were a threat to the male priests' monopoly on healing. Others were guilty of no more than being female and old. The symptoms are listed in the *Malleus Maleficarum,* the diagnostic manual of the day:

> All witchcraft comes from carnal lust which is in women insatiable … Three general vices appear to have special dominion over wicked women, namely, infidelity, ambition and lust. Therefore they are more than others inclined toward witchcraft who more than others are given to these vices.[22]

The Inquisition is a horrifically clear example of a well-organised programme of cruelty directed against those engaging in behaviours unacceptable or inconvenient to those in power. These programmes are often justified by theories disguising the violence as help for defective individuals. In the case of the murder of women diagnosed as witches the 'help' took the form of purifying their souls so they could enter heaven.

The return to science

The return to observation and reason known as the Renaissance was a gradual process. For instance, Johann Weyer (1515–1561) used observation in his relentless battle against the notion of witchery. He demonstrated that objects supposedly implanted by the Devil in the stomach of an accused woman carried no signs of gastric juices. For this he earned himself the diagnosis 'Weirus Insanus'.

Increased emphasis on the psychosocial origins of madness, the 'nurture' position, were reflected in Shakespeare's *Hamlet* and Cervantes' *Don Quixote*. Burton's *Anatomy of Melancholy* (1621), based partly on his need to understand his own chronic unhappiness, described one of the more popular diagnostic categories of this period. His theories were a blend of demonological and physiological. His treatments focused, like those of his contemporaries, on exercise, diets, drugs and, typical of the era, purgatives. He adds, however, a lovely description of one non-medical treatment for his own personal malady:

> It is the best thing in the world ... to get a trusted friend, to whom we may freely and sincerely pour out our secrets; nothing so delighteth and pleaseth the mind, as when we have a prepared bosom, to which our secrets

may descend, of whose conscience we are assured as our own, whose speech may ease our succourless estate, counsel relief, mirth expel our mourning, and whose very sight may be acceptable unto us.[23]

Such a therapeutic experience was seldom enjoyed by thousands of Europeans who, under the guise of medical treatment, were being locked away, worked, purged and drugged. Soon after its opening in 1656 the Hôpital Général in Paris was 'treating' 6,000 people. Typical of the view taken of this period by modern historians of psychiatry is the opinion that:

The Age of Reason marked a great leap forward. Through the efforts of the great scientists, philosophers, men of letters, and artists of the 17th century mental illness was further extricated from superstition and authoritarian error.[24]

However, on reflection, we think that the direction being adopted would turn out to be a transition from error based on one form of authority – religion, to error based on an equally dangerous form of authority – a particularly simplistic version, or perversion, of medical science.

Categorisation and confinement

From the latter part of the 17th century well into the 18th century the 'scientific' approach to understanding the world established the dominance it maintains today. During this 'Enlightenment', explanations of madness became dominated by categorisation and physiology. Psychological and social factors were buried under the relentless drive to discover *illnesses*. However, the Enlightenment's many attempts to find the imagined true categories of 'mental illness' led to no useful advances in physiological explanations.

Herman Boerhaave (1668–1738), for instance, justified continuation of blood-lettings and purgatives by discovering that 'melancholia' was caused by black juices. His invention of the rotating chair was more original. The theories used to portray this particular cruelty as a medical treatment varied. In Britain, Erasmus Darwin discovered that it reintroduced harmony to the 'disordered motions' of the nerves. Benjamin Rush, meanwhile, was convincing patients in North America that they were being strapped to a board and spun into unconsciousness to unclog their congested blood which, he had discovered, was the true cause of madness. The quest for specific brain pathology, still pursued today, was well under way. At London's Bethlem asylum John Haslem was already conducting autopsies.[25]

We might speculate as to how many of these people deemed 'mad' had died as a result of the poverty, neglect and violence endemic at the time. We might also note the enduring tendency to construct these human behaviours as theories about disordered brains rather the effects of social and economic conditions. Who were these mad people? The 1656 Edict which founded the Hôpital Général defined its population as: 'the poor of Paris, of both sexes, of all ages and from all localities, of whatever breeding and birth, in whatever state they may be, able-bodied or invalid, sick or convalescent, curable or incurable'.[26] The mad were locked away not for being mad but for being poor.

The 'Great Confinement', as Michel Foucault[27] describes this period, served the economic function of forcing inmates to work at a fraction of the going rate, under the guise of exercise or 'occupational therapy'. It served the political function of suppressing, under the guise of help for the poor and sick, the increasing number of uprisings amongst the unemployed. It also bolstered a moral belief in hard work. The Edict deemed that the major causes of all disorders were begging and idleness.

Moral treatment

Philippe Pinel in France, and William Tuke in England, are remembered for their humane treatment of mad people. Their approach, a good example of the religious position on the causes of mental health problems, has come to be known as 'Moral Treatment'.[28] Pinel, renowned for unchaining the insane, found it impossible to tell the difference between the effects of madness and the effects of cruel treatments in hospitals. Unlike many of the experts before them, Pinel and his fellow reformers were honest about their being in the business of imposing society's moral code on deviant individuals. Pinel was particularly concerned to eradicate celibacy, promiscuity, apathy and laziness. Such a morality was a special goal for women because: 'marriage constitutes for women a kind of preservative against the two sorts of insanity which are most inveterate and most often incurable'.[29]

Tuke founded the York Retreat in 1792 on the values of his Quaker upbringing. His son Samuel, who succeeded him, believed that 'to encourage the influence of religious principles over the mind of the insane is considered of great consequence as a means of cure'.[30] Patients would be invited to tea parties with the staff to assess their manners.

But Moral Treatment had little impact on the stranglehold of biological theories about madness. The categorisations and the quest for physical explanations continued. For instance, despite producing an important treatise on psychotherapy Johann Reil (1803) lumped together all silent patients into a single category, for which he prescribed the treatment of standing next to cannon fire.[31]

Aliens and alienists

The odd critical voice could be heard. Jean-Pierre Falret (1794–1870) went beyond Pinel's questions about the effects of cruel treatment and wondered whether the language being used might be similarly damaging. He suggested replacing 'mental disease' with 'mental alienation'. He was drawing attention to the processes by which we can become disconnected from other people and from society as a whole. He renamed those trying to help people reconnect 'alienists'. The medical profession were unimpressed.

History in a nutshell

To summarise, there seem to be at least four themes, rules if you like, about how society tends to respond to 'madness'.

1. 'Treatments' often seem to have the effect of suppressing behaviours, thoughts or feelings that are unacceptable to the majority or to those in power.

2. Those treatments have frequently been unhelpful and sometimes blatantly damaging.

3. There always seems to be experts who will argue that these ineffective or damaging treatments are actually for the good of the individual, who is seen as defective or abnormal in some way and in need of 'help'.

4. The way we think about people who are very distressed seems to always be contaminated by our tendency to want to separate 'them' from 'us', to exaggerate the differences

between the 'abnormal' and the 'normal', the 'mad' and 'the sane'. For centuries this even involved locking them away somewhere out of sight in places that symbolised our fear of insanity, of difference.

For those of you interested in the history of mental health issues, some more readings are suggested below. For now we hope we have shown that there has always been a range of explanations competing for our attention. So any debates you have been having with yourself, or others, about whether you were born with your problems or acquired them along the way (or a bit of both), and about how responsible you, or your family, friends or clients are for causing them, have been going on for centuries. That may, or may not, be reassuring. But you are certainly not alone in your wonderings.

This chapter is based on Chapter 2 of *Models of Madness* (Read, J, Mosher, LR & Bentall, R (eds) (2004) Hove: Brunner-Routledge).

Chapter 3
The 20th century and beyond:
The illness model

When a police officer asked a drunken man why he was peering at the ground around a lamp post, he said that he was looking for his keys. It was obvious that there were no keys on the pavement so the officer asked why the man was looking for them under the street lamp when he must have dropped them somewhere else. The man explained that he was looking under the street lamp because the light was better there.

History unfolds

The age-old nature vs. nurture debate continued into the 20th century. Up to the 1950s, the idea that psychological distress and disturbance were caused by 'nature' continued to be pursued by dedicated biological researchers supporting the professional structures of doctors and scientists whose interests lay in the 'medical model'. Initially, just about the only arguments for the 'nurture' side of the debate were presented by Sigmund Freud's psychoanalytic theory. However, from roughly the middle of the 20th century, the emerging field of social and behavioural science began to gain ground. Though at odds with Freud on the majority of points of philosophy and theory, the new science of behaviourism championed by John B. Watson and Frederick B. Skinner became the standard-bearer for the nurture point of view. Human psychology – personality, motives and behaviour, both how they developed and how they fell apart – was considered to be developed through interaction with the environment, rather than inborn. The behavioural science perspective on mental distress infused the mid-20th century with a new enthusiasm for looking for a cause of mental distress. Behaviourists' experiments (see Chapter 7) had shown that much of human behaviour is caused by 'reinforcement'.[1,2]

On the nature side of the debate, treatment successes were claimed for both lobotomies and electroshock treatment, but subsequent scrutiny raised questions about their effectiveness. The enduring problem for the nature argument at the time was that in order to explain their apparent treatment successes, biological psychiatry could only come up with either sweeping generic 'illness' theories on the one hand or speculative idiosyncratic theories on the other.

In the early 1950s the history of searching for explanations for mental distress took a path which has dictated the discourse right up to the present day. The pharmaceutical industry and a psychotechnology dedicated to increasing the medicalisation of life have created an endless array of 'illnesses' and 'disorders' with an attendant array of new drugs to 'cure' them. Our search for causes is inextricably intertwined with this development. We have to pause and ask 'What is it that we are trying to understand the cause of?' We ask this now because in the few words since the beginning of Chapter 1 we have covered several thousand years of attempts to understand disturbance and distress. In that period there have been times when the overarching explanations have changed ('religion', 'reason', and so on), but in the 20th century a new way of looking at human behaviour in general, including distress, began to dominate Western societies. In our attempt to understand the world we have brought scientific methods to bear in our search for meaning. This is not necessarily a problem, unless it is applied with a particularly peculiar twist: the tendency to see everything in *medical* terms – all behaviour becomes medicalised.

In the 1970s CAT (computerised axial tomography) and MRI (magnetic resonance imaging) scans helped scientists create visual representations of the human brain as it worked. These increasingly sophisticated techniques were pressed into service to look at the working brains of people diagnosed with different 'mental illnesses' to see if there was any difference in structure or function between the brain of a 'normal' person and a person with a 'mental illness'.

The potential of these and other emerging neuroimaging techniques for revealing brain structure and function led to President George W. Bush declaring the 1990s 'The Decade of the Brain' to 'enhance public awareness of the benefits to be derived from brain research.[3] It was to be a public and privately funded collaborative research initiative involving, amongst other institutions and agencies, the National Institutes of Health and the National Institute of Mental Health. In the search for causes the spotlight was turned on brain structure and function via these exciting new technologies.

The most recent scientific innovation to touch our search for causes was the Human Genome Project[4] launched in 1990, and coming to fruition with the complete genome published in 2003.

So the vast majority of research into the causes of mental health problems undertaken in the second half of the century was into either genes or brains. In a 2008 analysis it was found that for every study into the social causes of psychosis, for instance, there were 15 into biological factors.[5] Many of the brain researchers seemed not to understand that brain differences between two groups of people (e.g., depressed and happy) revealed by neuroimaging techniques, tell us absolutely nothing about the causes of mental health problems. This is because the brain (which has evolved specifically to interact with, and be changed by, the environment) responds to depressing things happening. So if you look at someone's brain after a loved one has died it will indeed look different from the brain of someone who has just fallen in love (and from the same person's brain at other times in their life). The essential question remains unanswered – which has caused the sadness: the bereavement or a collection of neurotransmitters? Indeed, not only is the question unanswered, but we maintain that it is unanswerable when asked from the poles of the nature–nurture debate. It is a complex system of interactions between events in the world and neurochemistry. There is, however, no need to have a 'chicken and egg' debate. In this instance the sadness was initially precipitated by an event in the world which caused a cascade of internal responses, *one* of which was neural activity, leading the person to feel 'down'. A natural, reasonable, indeed healthy response to an event in the world. And we must remember to be very careful how we understand what is a 'healthy' and 'unhealthy' (normal/abnormal, sane/insane) response in any given situation.

It has been shown that all the unusual features of the brains of people diagnosed 'schizophrenic' (frequently described as a brain disease) are found in the brains of young children who have been severely traumatised.[6]

The drive to medicalise more and more behaviours led researchers to make claims about more and more 'illnesses' and 'disorders' – not only for 'mental illnesses' but for just about every facet of human life, from gambling to unemployment, from being overweight to criminality, from shyness to alcoholism. Many of the studies claiming to find the gene for this or that were later called into question or proved to be simply wrong, but by then we had read headlines like 'Schizophrenia Genes Identified', which is a far better story than 'Follow up Studies Fail to Reproduce Findings of Earlier Study'. In 2008 an *American Journal of Psychiatry* paper,[7] described by the Editor as 'The most comprehensive genetic association study of genes previously reported to contribute to the susceptibility to schizophrenia' (i.e., a review of all previous studies) found 'nothing outside of what would be expected by chance'.[8]

As early as the 1960s and early 1970s there was some excellent research on the family's contribution to mental health problems and to the role of broader social factors like poverty (more about this in Chapter 6). A solution, or the appearance of a solution, to these two competing models – nature vs. nurture, biology vs. social factors – emerged.

The 'biopsychosocial' model

In the 1970s an integration of the two models was attempted. It became known as the 'biopsychosocial' approach and could also be called the 'stress-vulnerability' model. The idea was that we each have a varying degree of vulnerability to depression, distress, disturbance, madness etc. and that this vulnerability is then triggered by social stressors like poverty, neglect, violence etc. This model assumes, for example, that depressing events by themselves are not enough to make us *very* depressed – only those of us with a genetically inherited predisposition to get depressed or some other constitutional vulnerability (maybe due to mother's poor diet or smoking during pregnancy) will respond to those events with extreme depression. The greater your inherited or constitutional vulnerability the smaller the stress needed to tip you over the edge. This sounds like a good idea, giving equal weight to biology and the social environment – nature and nurture. The problem, however, is that because of the dominance of biological thinking it was assumed that the vulnerability *had* to be inherited genetically. This reduced social factors like child abuse, unemployment, loss, poor living conditions etc. to mere triggers of an underlying genetic or constitutional time bomb – only people who had the supposed genetic predisposition would become depressed, alcoholic, mad etc. It implied that social factors by themselves cannot cause mental health problems. This was both inaccurate and unhelpful, but it provided the illusion of an integration and many researchers and mental health professionals still refer to this model without realising that the vulnerability side of the equation can itself be caused by bad things happening during childhood. For example, if you are abused or neglected as a child you are more vulnerable to stresses (especially similar ones) later in life. Although we are, of course, born with genetic variations (including, quite probably, differences in our general sensitivity to stress) you don't need a genetic predisposition for bad things happening to overwhelm you, make you depressed or drive you crazy.

Better solutions to the nature–nurture debate

So, we think the biopsychosocial, or stress-vulnerability, attempt to resolve the debate is only helpful if we acknowledge that the vulnerability side of the equation can be caused by both our genetic makeup *and* the social environment we grow up in.

We now know, however, that just about everything we do, think or feel as human beings is partly determined by nature (our genes, brains etc.) and partly by nurture (our upbringing, current circumstances etc.). Some researchers have pointed out that it is, moreover, impossible to ever calculate what percentage of a given behaviour or problem, e.g., depression, is due to genetics and how much to the environment.[9] They point out that genes have no influence whatsoever without an environment and vice versa. They further remind us that as soon as the first cell divides in the developing embryo it has an environment. So where, they ask, does biology end and the environment begin? They just cannot be separated in the way that many well-intentioned researchers have tried to do in the past. After reviewing the science, Richard Bentall summarises our position concisely when he writes:

> Finally, substantial resources have been spent, and continue to be spent, in the attempt to discover the genetic origins of mental illness, whereas its social origins continue to be neglected. ... In this context it is important to note that no patient, not a single one, has ever benefited from genetic research into mental illness ... Indeed, from the point of view of patients, there can be few other areas of medical research that have yielded such a dismal return for effort expended.[10]

It seems that the whole genes vs. environment debate, which has been going on for centuries, is ill-directed and a waste of time in terms of coming up with a single identifiable cause. The two sets of factors are constantly interacting in an extremely complex way that is almost impossible to get a handle on if simple answers are what you're after. To complicate matters further, recent discoveries in 'epigenetics' (the study of how genes interact with their environment) have shown that the genes can be turned on and off by environmental factors.[11,12] Having the debate, even though it might seem sometimes overly academic and out of touch, has, however, taught us just how complex really useful explanations are likely to be. Neither side of the debate should be dismissed if we truly want to understand the causes of psychological distress.

We think the best way forward is to stop trying to figure out whether 19% or 32% of depression, or 'schizophrenia', is genetically determined and focus instead on determining the effect of factors that we can actually do something about. We don't think it's too helpful to turn the spotlight on genetic factors since recent history is laden with examples of how we have handled this idea poorly. We expect the vast majority of readers would agree that we don't want to return to the days of compulsory sterilisations conducted in the USA, Scandinavia and Germany in the 1930s to try to eliminate the supposed genes from the gene pool.[13] But a version of this still occurs in the USA today in the guise of 'genetic counselling' to encourage some people not to have babies. If poverty, child abuse etc., are causes of something (with or without a genetic predisposition to that thing) then we and many others argue that it is far more useful to focus on those and to do something to prevent them.[14]

This argument applies just as much to everyone's efforts to understand the cause of their own problems as it does at a societal level. You might be reading this book because you want to understand the causes of your problems a little better, or maybe you want to learn about the causes of psychological disturbance in general. You might also be reading this book because you actually want to do something about those problems. Of course having a new understanding can sometimes make a big difference all by itself – especially if someone has compounded their problems by blaming themselves or calling themselves 'ill', with the inevitable implication that they can do nothing to change.

But sometimes for things to get better we have to take our new understandings and actually use them to do something different. So, can you do anything about a person's genetic makeup? Can you do anything about the effects of a lonely or scary childhood, about a stressful work situation, about a bullying family member? What we are trying to say here is that spending time thinking, or worrying, about how much of a person's problem has been inherited is not going to get us very far. If we are looking at causes because we are really trying to find solutions, we think it is better to look towards those factors which it is more likely we can have an effect on.

The brain and biology

But what about the brain in all this? A lot of information leaflets and websites, often funded by drug companies,[15,16,17] will tell you that you have a chemical imbalance or some other 'brain abnormality'. This is one of the common arguments of those who see distress as an 'illness' and believe that specific brain differences show that nature is more important than nurture. But as we have already seen above, the idea that brain differences imply an illness or disease does not necessarily hold up. What use would a brain be if it did not respond to the environment? So it would be only natural for your brain to be, and possibly appear on neuroimaging scans to be, different when you are very anxious, or very depressed. It is another thing to say that those brain changes are *the cause* of the anxiety or depression.

Disease-centred versus drug-centred explanations

A disease-centred explanation

This argument, that complex, distressing experiences labelled as 'depression' or 'schizophrenia' and so on are illnesses caused by chemical imbalances in the brain, is often used by biologically oriented folk in the mental health field.

In order to make this claim they usually work backwards from the finding that the drugs used to try and help with the problem change certain chemical processes in the brain. The argument goes that if drug X lessens some of the symptoms of the experiences labelled as 'depression', and we know that drug X increases the levels of chemical Y in the brain, then depression *is caused by* a deficit of chemical Y. So in the real world it was noticed that, for example, paroxetine (trade names, Seroxat, Paxil) affects pathways in the brain by increasing the level of the neurotransmitter serotonin. Taking paroxetine appears to reduce a range of symptoms associated with the diagnosis of 'depression'. Therefore low levels of the neurotransmitter serotonin must cause a range of symptoms including depression.

This is known as a disease-centred model because it hinges upon the idea that a disease process causes the chemical imbalance that is subsequently relieved or restored by the drug. We will look at the evidence for this model later in this chapter. In her book *A Straight Talking Introduction to Psychiatric Drugs* in this series, British psychiatrist Joanna Moncrieff points out that the logic of the argument is similar to saying that since we notice that an alcoholic drink helps people overcome their inhibitions and be more socially outgoing, then that proves that shyness (or the condition labelled 'social anxiety disorder') is caused by a lack of alcohol in the brain. Or that since we notice that aspirin relieves headaches, that headaches are caused by a lack of aspirin in the bloodstream. Moncrieff suggests, instead, a drug-centred model to explain the effects of psychoactive medications.

A drug-centred explanation

Note that although we have used the example of paroxetine and depression, the models and their respective logic hold true for practically all diagnoses and psychoactive drugs (e.g., the relationship between the symptoms of the experience diagnosed as 'schizophrenia', levels of the neurotransmitter dopamine and the drug chlorpromazine).

A drug-centred explanation would say that psychoactive drugs act by inducing a state of intoxication which might either help the person taking the drug, make them feel worse, give them some relief of symptoms but with some unpleasant side effects or have no noticeable effect. The drug-centred model is so called because it focuses on the drug and doesn't create the notion that there is an illness which the drug is directly affecting, rebalancing or curing. In the drug-centred model, the relationship between the symptoms and the drug's action might:

1. have some *systematic* elements (affecting all people in much the same way) by virtue of what we know about the physiology of the drug's effects, but

2. will always have some *idiosyncratic* benefits or drawbacks as well (affecting individual people positively or negatively in unpredictable ways)

Using the same examples that we used in the section on disease-centred models, we can see that alcohol intoxication has the general side effect of disinhibition (taking away inhibitions), so the welcome effect on helping shyness and social anxiety is a specific action of the drug, but we do not think that it *cures* shyness. Similarly, we know that aspirin has a general analgesic (painkilling) effect – in particular it helps toothache and headache. However, no one believes that aspirin *cures* headache or toothache by rebalancing chemicals in the head or getting rid of infection in the teeth.

So a drug-centred model is accepted by many people as the real mechanism by which many drugs exert their beneficial effects. We are not alone in thinking that it is at least as good a model for understanding drug action as proposing that psychoactive drugs are actually correcting imbalances in neurotransmitters or other chemicals.

The reason we have gone into so much detail about *treatment* methods here is because theories about *causes* grow from post hoc (after the event) observations about what works. Sometimes these are helpful and even turn out to be correct. Sometimes they are unhelpful and send searches for causes up cul-de-sacs whilst wasting valuable time and resources on the false trails. What do you think?

Examples of theories of neurochemical malfunction
It is widely thought that brain chemicals called neurotransmitters contribute to the development of distressing experiences. In particular, the neurotransmitters serotonin and norepinephrine appear to play key roles. Originally, it was thought that low levels of these chemicals in the brain caused depression, but further research suggested that it is more complicated than that. More evidence encouraged some scientists to think that these two chemicals might regulate other neurotransmitters, such as dopamine and acetylcholine, that might also contribute to depression.[18,19] Later, the hormone melatonin was thought to play a role in depression. In winter, the decrease in sunlight causes the human body to produce more melatonin, which results in greater fatigue and the need to sleep more.[20] Some people are affected more strongly by this production of melatonin, resulting in what is called seasonal affective disorder (SAD),[21,22] leading to the idea that SAD is a form of depression.

This short excursion into a fragment of the research into neurotransmitters and 'mood' demonstrates that when we delve into brain function to see what possible explanations there might be to involve neurotransmitters in symptoms associated with various psychiatric diagnoses, the situation is not at all clear. We pretty soon find out how little is actually known about the detail of how what we think might happen in the brain is translated into lived experience. Getting one person's experience to match a picture generated by a brain scan is difficult enough, but it then becomes clear that to an important extent, everyone is different!

Nevertheless, it is possible to hypothesise what problems might be occurring. If we continue with the diagnosis of depression as our example, there could be:

- low levels of production of serotonin by brain cells

- a normal level of serotonin may be being made, but there could be a lack of receptor sites able to receive the serotonin that is made

- a problem preventing serotonin from reaching the receptor sites

- a shortage of the chemical from which serotonin is made (this is known as a precursor' and in the case of serotonin is a common substance called tryptophan found in many foods)

If any of these neurochemical problems occur, theorists suggest it could lead to depression. In addition, theorists think that serotonin pathways might be implicated in obsessive-compulsive behaviour and anxiety. Indeed anxiety is also seen by many as the key driver to many symptoms associated with mood problems, so this is not an unusual suggestion. However, it also demonstrates just how complex and interconnected the brain systems are – we can pretty soon come to the conclusion that serotonin is linked to everything and then the hypothesis loses its predictive power.

Although it is widely believed that a lack of serotonin plays a role in depression, there are currently no techniques to measure serotonin levels in the living brain. It follows that there have not been any studies *proving* that brain levels of serotonin – or any other neurotransmitter for that matter – are in short supply when depression (or indeed any diagnosable *mental illness*) occurs. However, blood levels of serotonin are measurable and there is some evidence to show that they are lower in people who suffer from depression.[23] Amongst the several problems with such findings (not least the disputes about whether they can be repeated) we find that it still can't be shown whether or not the claimed low serotonin causes the symptoms of depression, or the depression causes serotonin levels to drop.

So both the evidence and the theories of neurochemical involvement in depression are, to say the least, incomplete and should be considered works in progress. It is really difficult to pin down straightforward relationships between neurochemical events and experiences.

Finally, you may have noticed that we slipped in the above paragraphs the fact that the precursor for serotonin is tryptophan. We did this so we could show how a very wide range of explanations and theories can spring up from rather scant and unreliable evidence. In the first place it is an undisputed fact that tryptophan is the precursor to serotonin. Serotonin is effectively made from tryptophan. Tryptophan, however is not manufactured in the body – it is an 'essential' amino acid – we have to eat foods which contain it. And this fact gives rise to theories that experiences which are likely to be diagnosed as depression can be affected by the amount of tryptophan in the diet. In simple terms: eat more tryptophan and you'll cheer up. Indeed a quick Internet search turned up a website selling alternative cures for tinnitus with the following quote:

> Most of us know, I believe, that it's the tryptophan in
> turkey that promotes the sense of well-being we associate
> with Thanksgiving. ... Decreased serotonin levels play a
> key role in the development of depression. The only source
> for serotonin in the brain is tryptophan. It cannot be
> converted from any other substance. If there is not enough
> tryptophan in the diet, it can lead to anxiety and
> depression.[24]

There are, of course, many explanations of why someone
might have a feeling of well-being after eating turkey that
are more plausible than the amount of tryptophan it
contains! It turns out that tofu, cod, cheese and pork all
contain more tryptophan than turkey. We can see, though,
how human imagination, set free from the discipline of
scientific evidence, can come up with explanations which
have superficial plausibility. The jury is out, not only on the
mood-lifting properties of tofu and turkey, but on the
particular role of serotonin in depression as well.

Can drugs cause psychosis?

It has been known for thousands of years that certain
substances have a mood-altering effect and more recently we
have discovered a little about how this happens. Morphine,
cocaine, alcohol, caffeine, cannabis and psilocybin (found in
'magic' mushrooms) are just a few of the more well known
of these substances. The chances are that almost all readers
will have taken and therefore experienced the effects of one
or more of them. The effects of these substances are caused
by their action on neurotransmitter systems. Some
substances (e.g., alcohol) have an effect on many
neurotransmitter systems at once, and these effects can work
in complex ways, sometimes against each other:

- alcohol affects the dopamine system, making you feel excited

- alcohol affects the glutamate system causing muscle relaxation and slurred speech

- alcohol affects the gamma-aminobutyric acid system making you calm and drowsy

Other substances (e.g., morphine and cocaine) have a very discrete effect on one system only and have been called 'chemical scalpels' because they are so specific in their action that they can be used with precision in medical treatments.

When it comes to understanding distressing psychological symptoms, there is an inescapable logic in the idea that if some drugs appear to lessen distressing symptoms, then other drugs might exacerbate them, or even be able to cause them in the first place. It is also possible that some substances might throw neurotransmitter systems out of kilter, temporarily or permanently. Add to that the fact that the effects of using substances like cannabis and magic mushrooms are experienced as being very similar to some of the symptoms of psychoses, and it's easy to hypothesise possible links.

In statistical terms there is a demonstrably reliable relationship between cannabis use and psychosis, but this is not completely straightforward. Some readers will have personal experiences of, or know of others who have had, extremely unpleasant experiences after using cannabis. We know that cannabis is widely used in the Western world, particularly by adolescents – a time in people's lives which is particularly associated with the development of symptoms associated with a diagnosis of psychosis.[25] We also know that there is an association between cannabis use and the development of psychosis.[26] It's important to understand that an association between two things simply means that the two events are likely to occur together. It doesn't mean that one event causes the other. There are at least three logical possibilities in the case of cannabis and psychosis:

- cannabis use causes psychosis (we will look at some competing possibilities below)

- psychosis causes cannabis use (not as daft as it might seem, since we know that people will try all sorts of things to get rid of their symptoms, and alcohol and cannabis are high up on the list because some people find the effects calming or numbing)

- a third variable which we can't see is causing this association (an everyday example of this is the fact that there is an association between eating ice cream and drowning. Why is this? Because when the weather warms up, more people go swimming in the sea and ice cream is more popular. No one suggests that eating ice cream will cause you to drown!) It's worth remembering this type of 'association' because it's usually the kind of finding that lies behind news headlines 'linking' schizophrenia and other mental health problems with just about everything

The active ingredient in cannabis is tetrahydrocannabinol (THC), which attaches itself to the cannabinoid receptors (found in three areas of the brain) and in research terms there are several possible hypotheses that might explain the link between cannabis use and symptoms. These are, in short form:

- cannabis causes psychosis
- cannabis precipitates psychosis in people who are predisposed to it
- cannabis causes changes in the brain which make us more likely to respond to stress with symptoms of psychosis
- cannabis makes symptoms worse in people already suffering from unpleasant experiences when they try to alleviate them by using it
- cannabis causes temporary psychosis-like symptoms
- cannabis does not cause psychosis

If we look at a wide range of research, however, it's difficult to come to a firm conclusion on whether or not cannabis use causes symptoms associated with psychosis. A recent study tried to sort out the effects attributable to the use of cannabis and childhood sexual abuse on the rate of psychosis.[27] Readers will now appreciate some of the difficulties of working this out. Mark Shevlin and his colleagues looked at the development of symptoms in groups of people who had:

1. no sexual trauma or cannabis use (this is the reference group to which the other groups were compared – it gives a type of background level of diagnosis of psychosis)
2. sexual trauma with no cannabis use ever
3. cannabis use with no sexual trauma ever
4. first sexual trauma occurring before first cannabis use
5. first cannabis use occurring before first sexual trauma

They found that, in comparison to group 1, group 2 were a little more than twice as likely to receive a diagnosis of psychosis, whereas group 3 were no more likely to receive a diagnosis of psychosis than group 1. Group 4 were four times more likely to receive a diagnosis than group 1, and just about the same result was obtained for group 5. This was a complicated study which made adjustments for a number of factors so as to eliminate rogue effects.

From this study it looks as though on its own, cannabis use isn't a significant factor in the development of psychosis or psychotic-like symptoms. Childhood sexual abuse, however, is linked to the development of such symptoms and when combined with cannabis use, it seems to become a really strong factor. This seems to support our general theme in this book, namely that distressing experiences and symptoms which might be diagnosed as psychosis have many complex causes, both physical (biological/neurochemical), psychological (e.g., trauma or abuse) and social (e.g., poverty, unemployment).

In summary, drugs are consumed by people *because they have an effect* but it's difficult to predict what distressing effects there might be from person to person. Trauma at any time of life can result in distressing reactions, and trauma during childhood is very likely indeed to lead to adult symptoms and diagnoses of psychosis. Combining the two (whether or not the drugs are used as self-medication for the effects of trauma etc.) seems particularly potent and we should be arranging child protection, education and family support to take account of this.

Our conclusion is that whether we focus on genes or the brain, the nature–nurture argument is not very helpful in understanding the causes of our problems and virtually useless when it comes to figuring our what we can do about those problems. The remaining questions are: why do we as a society and as a mental health culture set by professionals, seem to prefer to base our understanding on such a polarised debate? And why is there such a bias towards the view that nature is far more important than nurture in causing our problems? Biologically oriented mental health professionals – mostly but not exclusively psychiatrists – promote this view for several possible reasons ranging from the understandable difficulty that some of them have to engage on a human level with very distressed or distressing people (preferring instead to keep their distance by just making a diagnosis and prescribing a drug), to a genuine belief that an illness explanation is more helpful because it avoids having to 'blame' anyone (see Chapter 5). Another influential group promote illness explanations for more obvious reasons.

The pharmaceutical industry

No discussion of what happened to our thinking about the causes of mental health problems in the second half of the 20th century would be complete without looking at the role of the pharmaceutical industry. Most discussions, however, ignore it completely. This is because, generally speaking, mental health researchers and professionals believe they are immune to economic and political pressures, that they are objective, scientific. We explained in Chapter 1 how we think it is practically impossible to be objective. We don't make this claim ourselves. We do, however, demand, and suggest everyone demands, transparency when it comes to vested interests in different types of explanation.

One of us (JR) was recently asked to write an article for a new journal in the psychosis field.[28] To encourage him to accept the invitation he was told that the journal is sent free to 20,000 psychiatrists in the USA. How are those 20,000 selected? According to which 20,000 have prescribed the most antipsychotic drugs in the preceding year!

Regardless of your position on the causes of mental health problems, most people now understand that the pharmaceutical industry has massive influence over mental health research, research journals, teaching institutions, professional organisations, drug-regulating authorities, the information we are offered over the Internet, and even (especially in the USA) the politicians and bureaucrats responsible for our mental health services. After decades of silence, more and more professionals who are concerned by this situation are beginning to speak out on this issue.[29,30,31]

One problem is that many researchers, research programmes, journals, and university departments and special interest groups have become dependant on drug company money.[32,33,34] The industry has particularly expanded its influence by funding the websites of community groups. Three recent studies show that in the areas of depression, post-traumatic stress disorder and schizophrenia about half of all websites are funded by the industry and that these sites are biased in favour of biological approaches to understanding and/or treating these conditions.[35,36,37] The pharmaceutical industry is enormously wealthy and enormously powerful, conducting more and better research on how to effectively market their products than psychologists do on evaluating psychological treatments or service providers do on evaluating medication-free mental health services.

It is interesting to note that some of those involved in the leading psychological approach at the end of the 20th century, cognitive therapy (see Chapter 7), have used their thought-monitoring and changing techniques to ensure patients take their medication. Treatment compliance is an important element of medical model therapies, so this type of cognitive therapy, 'Compliance Therapy', aims to do what it says on the tin.

This single-track approach means that fewer and fewer people are able to actively seek explanations for distress outside of a very narrow band of possibilities. It is difficult to obtain funding or approval for research into psychological and social explanations when our day-to-day understanding is flooded with medical metaphors for distress and just about every problem in living, however minor.

A new century

There are, of course, many exceptions to simplistic, illness approaches. Throughout the world during the last century, many mental health professionals continued trying to work on a human rather than a chemical level. Will the 21st century see more support for psychological explanations? Will the social causes of mental health problems finally be given the attention they deserve?

The situation was summarised when, in 2005, the President of the American Psychiatric Association, Dr Steven Sharfstein wrote:

> We must examine the fact that as a profession, we have allowed the bio-psycho-social model to become the bio-bio-bio model ... If we are seen as mere pill pushers and employees of the pharmaceutical industry, our credibility as a profession is compromised.[38]

Professor Mike Shooter, President of the Royal College of Psychiatrists in the UK, added:

> I cannot be the only person to be sickened by the sight of parties of psychiatrists standing at the airport desk with so

many perks about them that they might as well have the name of the company tattooed across their foreheads.[39]

The ever-increasing prescription rates for psychiatric drugs, especially for children and the elderly, do not give cause for optimism. By 2005 one in twenty men and one in nine women in the USA were taking antidepressants.[40] At the turn of the century there were 22 million prescriptions for antidepressants in the UK. By 2007 this had surged to 34 million.[41]

However there are some signs that psychosocial explanations have not disappeared altogether. If we look at the diagnosis of 'schizophrenia', since the 1990s many studies have shown that factors like poverty, urban living, child abuse, etc. are highly predictive of who ends up hearing voices or having delusions, with or without a genetic predisposition.[42,43]

An increasing number of psychiatric journals now have strict requirements about researchers declaring funding from, and conflicts of interest with, drug companies. One recently launched journal, *Psychosis: Psychological, Social and Integrative Approaches*,[44] refuses to take drug company advertising. Some governments and professional organisations have begun imposing restrictions on how much money psychiatrists (and other doctors) can receive from drug companies. The Norwegian Medical Association recently barred conference organisers from accepting drug company money if they want the conference to qualify as being 'educational'. Recent legislation has, at last, forced drug companies to disclose all of their studies into their drugs, not just the two or three that they chose to submit to drug regulation agencies (which naturally tended to be the studies that found the drug to be safe and effective). This has at last led to comprehensive, rather than highly selective, reviews of the research. One of these recently showed that antidepressants are, for the vast majority of recipients, no more effective than placebos (e.g., empty capsules).[45]

We finish with some warnings from neuroscientist Steven Rose, who outlines the dangers of looking for causes exclusively in an individual's biology:

> Consider the world-wide epidemic of depression identified by the World Health Organisation (WHO) as *the* major health hazard of this century, in the moderation – though scarcely cure – of which vast tonnages of psychotropic drugs are manufactured and consumed each year. Prozac is the best known ... Questions of why this dramatic rise in the diagnosis of depression is occurring are rarely asked – perhaps for fear it should reveal a malaise not in the individual but in the social and psychic order. Instead, the emphasis is overwhelmingly on what is going on within a person's brain and body. [46]

He continues:

> The neurogenetic-industrial complex thus becomes ever more powerful. Undeterred by the way that molecular biologists ... are beginning to row back from genetic determinist claims ... psychometricians ... behaviour geneticists ... and evolutionary psychologists are claiming genetic roots to areas of human belief, intentions and actions long assumed to lie outside biological explanation. Not merely such long-runners as intelligence, addiction and aggression, but even political tendency, religiosity and the likelihood of mid-life divorce are being removed from the province of social and/or personal psychological explanation into the province of biology. With such removal comes the offer to treat, to manipulate, to control.[47]

It will require all of us, users of mental health services and mental health staff, to work together to create sufficient conceptual space and financial resources to bring balance to the important task of seeking explanations for madness. Then together we can turn mental health services in the 21st century into ones where the first questions asked are not necessarily 'Which illness have you got?' and 'Are you taking your medication?' but 'What is troubling you?'; 'What do you think has happened to bring this about?'; and 'What do you need from us?'

Chapter 4
Can we understand causes through diagnoses and labels?

When someone comes into contact with mental health services as a patient they will probably be given a diagnosis of some sort. Many of us even try to diagnose ourselves (or our loved ones), often by surfing the Internet. Having a label to apply to our problems can be experienced as very helpful – at least we now have a word for what is happening to us (or, in medical terms, what illness we've got). It can sometimes also appear to give us an explanation. If there is a word that experts use to describe our difficulties then that suggests two things. Firstly, other people must have the same problems; and that can be very comforting. Secondly, we might assume that the experts who have come up with the name must know something about what causes it and how to 'treat' it. That can be even more reassuring.

Psychiatric diagnoses, however, are something of a mixed blessing. As well as looking at the pros and cons of diagnoses we will briefly outline the nature and history of diagnosing and describe how it works in practice today.

The human ability to categorise and label things in our world is fantastically helpful. It is practically 'natural' to us – one of the first thought processes we develop as human beings. It is completely understandable, therefore, that humans have always applied labels to distressing or unusual behaviour. In Chapter 2, for example, we came across 'hysterics', 'lunatics' and 'witches'. A comprehensive history would produce hundreds of terms, tried and discarded over the centuries – and that's just in one culture. The task facing us, and our predecessors, has always been the same: to lump together a set of behaviours and apply a name, in the hope that somehow this will increase our understanding.

There is a tradition in literature and the history of human ideas that suggests that whenever we can name something, it gives us power over it. So if we can name the disturbance or distress, we can categorise it and control it. This usually means putting it in a group with something that it appears to resemble and creating the illusion of a dividing line, in this case between the 'mad' and the 'normal'. The labels, which often sound a bit medical, a bit scientific, or at least a bit 'Latinish' – like 'melancholia' or 'dementia paranoides' – have sadly proved more effective at dividing 'us' from 'them' than increasing our understanding of what causes the problem in question.

As we have suggested, naming and categorising are essential for learning anything about the world, for storing the millions of bits of information that bombard us every day. Without being able to categorise, and thereby quickly recognise situations and people that are dangerous, we would not survive the first few years of life. So humans who do survive have become very good at categorising.

There are at least two problems, however, when we apply this skill to one another. Firstly, since our survival depends upon rapid categorisation, we all too quickly put people (including ourselves) in boxes and these labels tend to stick. Then we find we have put people into boxes from which they (we) can never escape. From that moment on we interpret everything they do through the filter of our understanding that they are an 'x' sort of person. Secondly, we tell ourselves that we now understand why a person does what they do, why they are who they are and so on: 'Of course they act like y because they are a y sort of a person.'

Or, in the case of psychiatric diagnoses, 'Of course they do "schizophrenic" things – they are "schizophrenic".' It is worth remembering that this whole construction of assumed 'understanding' has come about simply because we arbitrarily named it, and there is a huge difference between naming something and understanding it.

The important point here is that a diagnosis tells us *nothing* at all about what causes someone to act in a certain way. It is nothing more or less than an arbitrary label applied to a group of behaviours (or ways of thinking or feeling). This means that the reassurance gained from receiving a diagnosis, the belief that 'At least now I know what I've got and why I feel/act the way I do', is simply an illusion. All you really know is that a diagnosis is the word that experts use to *label* your behaviours, thoughts or feelings. They haven't understood it any better at all.

Although psychiatric diagnoses tell us nothing about the causes of mental health problems, it is notable that medical language (which tends to give it authority, even though there is still no understanding) is built into the 940-page *Diagnostic and Statistical Manual* (DSM), the book most commonly used around the world to help mental health professionals decide what diagnosis to apply.[1] Almost every diagnosis (itself a medical-sounding word) ends with 'disorder'. For example, it lists 'anxiety disorder', 'depressive disorder', 'personality disorder', 'panic disorder' etc. and, for our children, 'conduct disorder' 'attention deficit hyperactivity disorder' etc.). In this way our problems are made to *sound* like illnesses whether they are or not, especially when the behaviours used to decide which 'disorder' we have are called 'symptoms'.

The DSM itself acknowledges that it actually says nothing at all about causes, yet its medical language implies that what are being described are illnesses. This choice of language, consistent with the overarching term 'mental illness' is unsurprising given that the DSM is written by medical doctors (psychiatrists are trained as medical doctors before they specialise in psychiatry) from the country with one of the most biological approaches to mental health in the world (the USA).

It hasn't always been so. In the very first edition of the DSM, in 1952, the same problems now called 'disorders' were all called 'reactions'! This was a different era, in which psychoanalytic psychiatrists were in the ascendancy in the USA. Like the public (see Chapter 5) they understood that mental health problems stem largely from life events and our interpretations of those events, rather than from faulty genes or brain chemicals. The difference between believing that your difficulties are caused by your having some kind of disorder and believing that you are having an understandable reaction to your life history and circumstances is enormous.

This diagnostic approach to human distress medicalises all sorts of things, turning our reactions to life events into disorders. Feeling very sad after something sad has happened becomes Depressive Disorder, being very nervous without really knowing why becomes Generalized Anxiety Disorder. More and more problems have been redefined as 'disorders' or 'illnesses', supposedly caused by genetic predispositions and biochemical imbalances, with life events relegated to mere triggers of an underlying biological time bomb. Excessive gambling, drinking, drug use or eating are illnesses. So are eating, sleeping, and having sex too little. Being painfully shy has become 'Avoidant Personality Disorder'. Beating people up is now 'Intermittent Explosive Disorder'.

Our children are labelled too. Being bad at sums has become 'Mathematics Disorder'. Ignoring other people's feelings (once called being naughty) means your child is suffering from 'Conduct Disorder'. If this also includes getting angry with grownups the diagnosis changes to 'Oppositional Defiant Disorder'. A diagnosis much in the news recently (because of alarming increases in the prescribing of amphetamines) is 'Attention Deficit Hyperactivity Disorder'. The 'symptoms' of ADHD include: fidgeting, losing things, talking excessively, and difficulty playing quietly or taking turns.[2] Of course children sometimes have problems. But does the act of simply labelling them help in any way? Readers wanting to pursue this theme might find Sami Timimi's book in this series, *A Straight Talking Introduction to Children's Mental Health Problems,* interesting.[3]

Since this book is about the causes of mental health problems, we ask whether diagnostic labelling of behaviours (whatever their nuisance value to other people) actually takes us any nearer to understanding the cause of the behaviour. We think the answer is quite simply 'no'. Furthermore we are concerned that such labelling, with its apparent scientific basis, sometimes conceals the *actual* causes by locating the problem entirely within the child. From such a viewpoint there appears to be no value in prevention programmes. We just need to medicate the 'sick' child.

This locating of the problem entirely in the individual is just one of the many downsides of a diagnostic/labelling/categorising approach to assessing mental health problems. A diagnostic approach also graces someone's arbitrary idea with a baseless 'scientific' authority. A diagnosis also, by giving the impression that something is actually known about this behaviour, means that we stop looking for real explanations. The diagnosis itself, however arbitrary, substitutes for real explanation and understanding. These issues are dealt with in detail in another book in this series, by British psychologist Richard Bentall. But to introduce the two vital, if rather academic, issues of 'reliability' and 'validity' here are a couple of quotes from Richard's earlier writing:

On reliability:[4]

> A wide range of evidence suggests that our current system of diagnostic classification has led psychiatry down a path that is no more scientific than astrology. Like star signs, psychiatric diagnoses are widely believed to tell us something specific about ourselves, to explain our behaviour and personality, and to predict what will happen to us in the future. Like star signs, diagnoses fail on   all of these counts.[5]

On validity:[6]

> Even if the reliability problem were one day solved, there would be no guarantee that the resulting diagnoses would be scientifically valid or clinically useful. If a disease is operationally defined in terms of an arbitrary but unrelated set of criteria a meaningless diagnosis can be assigned to patients with a high degree of reliability. This would be the case if, for example, we defined 'Bentall's Disease' in terms of such easily defined symptoms as hair colour, the number of summer colds experienced in the last five years, and the number of Pink Floyd albums owned.[7]

Bentall is by no means the first to point out these problems. Thirty-five years ago researchers found that when 134 US and 194 British psychiatrists were given a description of a patient, 69% of the US psychiatrists diagnosed 'schizophrenia', but only 2% of the British psychiatrists did so. The majority of the British psychiatrists (75%) said the

Advantages and disadvantages of the diagnostic approach to understanding mental health problems

Advantages

- *Assists communication* (about research and treatment)

- *Brings relief* (through appearance of an explanation, and awareness that others have the same problem)

- *Assists managers/policy makers* decide whose problems are serious enough to deserve treatment/ funding

Disadvantages

- *Locates problem entirely in individual*

- *Suggests an illness – ignores social causes*

- *Underestimates capacity for change*

- *Reduces hope of recovery*

- *Stigma from labelling*

- *Categories vs. dimensions* ('pigeon-holing' vs. acknowledging that most of us have the problem to varying degrees at different times)

- *Poor reliability* (experts can't agree about who has got what)

- *Poor validity* (diagnoses don't predict future or our response to treatment)

- *'Co-morbidity'* (most of us have two, three, four or more DSM 'disorders')

person had a 'personality disorder', a view held by just 7% of their USA colleagues.[8]

The absurdity of all this was illustrated by a famous study in which 'normal' people, admitted to psychiatric hospitals after saying they heard the words 'empty' or 'thud', were all diagnosed 'schizophrenic'. None of the staff, but many of the patients, recognised that the 'pseudo-patients' were 'normal'. A follow-up study, in which hospital staff were told that 'pseudo-patients' would be admitted, produced a 21% detection rate by staff. But no 'pseudo-patients' had been admitted![9] American psychologist Lauren Slater considers this study one of the 'great psychological experiments of the 20th century' and has recently conducted a small repeat version of it – with similar results.[10]

By 1992, researchers had identified 16 systems of classifying schizophrenia. Out of 248 patients the number diagnosed as schizophrenic by these systems ranged from 1 to 203.[11]

Conclusions

We make no apologies for repeating ourselves (again!) in this conclusion. The power of the labels we use in everyday life is huge, especially when we invest the person or institution doing the labelling with any authority. And when we, the labelled, are in a position of weakness and vulnerability (we are terrified and desperate for help) the process becomes very hard to challenge. A further problem is that since the whole of life is becoming medicalised, we fail to notice the flimsy reliability and validity of the labels. It has become a given, taken for granted – a fact about the world that we can only think from, rather than think about. French sociologist Pierre Bourdieu captures it when he says: 'it goes without saying because it comes without saying'.[12] Furthermore, any critical voices are easily dismissed (labelled, or 'diagnosed') as 'antipsychiatry', irresponsible, troublemaking, dangerous, unscientific or radical.

The main point of all this, in a book about causes of mental health problems, is that, contrary to what we might hope, a psychiatric diagnosis doesn't help us understand what is going on at all. And if we swallow the idea that we 'have' some sort of 'disorder' or 'illness' inside us, the diagnosis cannot only mask the real causes of our problems – which we, and many others argue, lie in the events and circumstances of our lives. Furthermore, such acceptance of the power of diagnosis disempowers us since it can discourage our belief that we can do anything to make things better ourselves. After all if you are one of those people who happen to 'have' a 'depressive disorder' (in your brain or your genes) then there isn't too much you can really do about it (other than take medication for life). But if you realise that your sometimes feeling depressed is largely a reaction to depressing things happening then maybe, with help if necessary, you can do something to avoid more depressing things happening or to change how you are reacting to them.

If you like having a label to sum up all the complexities of what is happening to you, then hang on to your diagnosis for all you are worth. If, on the other hand, you want to try figuring out where the problem actually started and what is maintaining it, and are even willing to try something new in an effort to make things better, then it's probably best not to pay too much attention to your diagnosis. And of course, you can always do both if that's what works best for you, since it's not just a slogan when we say everyone is different and requires a unique approach. It's a fact.

Chapter 5
Public opinion: Depression is caused by depressing things happening

While we experts continue to argue about the causes of mental health problems, the public have already voted. In research surveys all over the world the result is the same: the vast majority of lay people, the people in the street, think that social causes explain mental distress (however severe or enduring) better than biological causes.

John begins many of his international lectures with a slide showing all the countries where the public have been found to believe that things like poverty, family stress, loneliness, relationship problems, child abuse, etc. are more important causes of mental illness than factors like heredity or chemical imbalances. He does this because in some quarters of the mental health field, such views, and especially research about child abuse being a cause of psychosis, are dismissed as 'extreme', 'dangerous' or 'naïve'. Some mental health professionals still think that the idea that bad things happen and screw us up is very controversial. So he says, 'Instead of bringing a support group with me I have brought several million people, from 16 countries, who agree with me. The research findings I will present to you today are only controversial to a numerically tiny sector of the mental health world – biological psychiatrists.'

The list on the slide behind him while he talks is: Australia, China, England, Ethiopia, Germany, Greece, India, Ireland, Italy, Japan, Malaysia, Mongolia, Russia, South Africa, Turkey, and the USA.[1]

Most of these surveys allow respondents to choose more than one explanation rather than just choose between social and biological. Often there is quite a long list of possible causes to choose from. This reveals that the public actually hold a quite sophisticated approach to the causes of mental health problems. They certainly recognise both social and biological causes, adopting what the experts would call a 'multifactorial' approach. There is, however, a very strong pattern in terms of what sorts of causes they think are most important. In all 16 countries social causes easily beat biological illness-type causes.

We'll look at just a few of the many studies demonstrating that the public understand that human distress is primarily caused by our social environment. Some surveys ask about the causes of mental health problems in general and others focus on the causes of specific problems, usually either depression or 'schizophrenia'.

In England, a 1997 survey found, in relation to mental health in general, that 'Life events, family problems and economic hardship were mentioned frequently, with genetic and biological causes noted much less frequently.'[2] When Londoners were asked more specifically about schizophrenia: 'Overall subjects seemed to prefer environmental explanations referring to social stressors and family conflicts – e.g., "being mercilessly persecuted by family and friends" and "having come from backgrounds that promote stress".'[3] Another London study found that the most endorsed causal model of schizophrenia was 'unusual or traumatic experiences or the failure to negotiate some critical stage of emotional development', followed by 'social, economic, and family pressures'.[4] 'It seems that lay people have not been converted to the medical view and prefer psychosocial explanations.'[5] 'Subjects agreed that schizophrenic behaviour had some meaning and was neither random nor simply a symptom of an illness.'[6]

An Irish survey found that the most commonly cited causes for the positive symptoms of schizophrenia (e.g., hallucinations and delusions) were stressful life events. Only 11% cited biogenetic causes. For negative symptoms (e.g., social withdrawal) the most frequently cited cause was childhood problems such as 'lack of adequate parental love'.[7] Only 5% cited biogenetic causes.

A 2004 survey of Australians[8] found that the most likely cause of depression was 'day-to-day-problems such as stress, family arguments, difficulties at work or financial difficulties', which was endorsed as a likely cause by 97% of Australians. A close second was 'the recent death of a close friend or relative' (96%), followed by 'traumatic events' (94%) and 'problems from childhood such as being badly treated or abused, losing one or both parents when young or coming from a broken home' (92%). The highest biological-type explanation was 'inherited or genetic' (67%). Although 'schizophrenia' is said, by biological psychiatrists, to be the most biologically based of all their supposed 'illnesses', the public in Australia (and all over the world) disagrees. The pattern was the same as for depression. The top four causes were the same four social causes listed above, with 'inherited or genetic' a distant fifth.

The most comprehensive series of large-scale national surveys has been conducted, over many years, in Germany. In 2005 the researchers responsible reviewed all their studies and concluded that, for both depression and schizophrenia, 'acute stress in the form of life events is the most frequently endorsed cause, followed by chronic stress in partnership and family'.[9]

'Patients'

Since people who use mental health services are members of the public, it should come as no surprise that they also understand their problems in terms of what has gone on in their lives more so than in terms of genes and neurotransmitters. Recently, numerous books[10,11,12] and journal articles[13,14] have ended decades of disinterest in what people diagnosed with psychotic disorders like 'schizophrenia' have to say about their own experiences and what might have caused them. While a vast array of causes are cited, showing again that everyone is different, many write about pretty bad childhood experiences that they believe contributed to their difficulties in adulthood.

A 2005 US study of four 'stakeholder groups' concluded, in relation to 'schizophrenia', that 'Of the factors consistent with a non-biomedical view of mental illness, consumers [service users], family members, and the general public consistently endorsed these as causes more frequently than did the clinicians' (68%).[15] Consumers were the most likely (66%), and clinicians the least likely (18%), to cite 'the way he was raised' as a cause. Clinicians were significantly more likely to endorse genetics as a cause than the other three groups, and consumers were less likely than clinicians to endorse chemical imbalance. 'Stressful circumstances' was cited significantly more often by both consumers and family members than by clinicians.

Other studies of the causal explanations held by people diagnosed with schizophrenia find strong psychosocial beliefs, in both Germany[16] and England.[17] The causes espoused as 'likely/very likely' by Germans who experience psychosis were: 'recent psychosocial factors' – 88%, 'personality' – 71%, 'family' – 64% and 'biology' – 31%. Indeed the German 'patients' endorsed 'psychosocial stress factors' even more strongly than the rest of the population. A recent study in London found that only 5% of people diagnosed as 'schizophrenic' believed that their problems were a result of having a 'mental illness' and only 13% cited other biological causes, but 43% cited social causes such as interpersonal problems, stress and childhood events. (Members of ethnic minorities within the sample were even less likely than their white counterparts to endorse biological causes.)[18]

A sensible response to these findings might be 'well, they should know'. But 'Not at all!' say some psychiatrists. Their believing that they have been driven mad by awful things happening to them is still sometimes dismissed as a lack of 'insight' into the fact that they have an 'illness'. Some psychiatrists even use this supposed lack of insight as a diagnostic indicator that their 'patients' are still ill. To be seen as recovered, it seems, a person has to admit that they were wrong to think that their problems are related to their life circumstances. They have to agree with the psychiatrist's opinion that they have a biologically based illness. This is a great example of how dominant the 'medical model' has become. The original (psychoanalytic) meaning of 'insight' was in fact the ability to understand your current difficulties in relation to past life events, especially those in childhood. Now it means, for some psychiatrists, exactly the opposite.

Family members

If one were to rely entirely on the Internet and the media to find out what the relatives of people who use mental health services think, you might conclude that most family members strongly endorse the illness model and want to see their 'sick' relatives permanently on medication or kept in hospital. It turns out that the so-called 'family organisations', which are often quoted or have representatives on news and current affairs programmes, are heavily sponsored by drug companies. Organisations such as SANE in the UK, NAMI (National Alliance for the Mentally Ill) in the USA, and the Schizophrenia Society of Canada, which receive so much media coverage, are not at all representative of family members in general.[19]

We have already mentioned the 2005 USA study that showed that both consumers and their relatives have, like the general public, a far more psychosocial framework than mental health professionals. Numerous other studies have shown that relatives of mental health service users elsewhere in the world also share the same beliefs as the general public. This is true even for that supposedly biological illness 'schizophrenia'. As early as 1988 the German researchers mentioned earlier cited five international studies showing that the relatives of 'schizophrenics' believed that the causes were social. They went on to repeat the finding among German relatives.[20] A more recent Italian survey of 709 relatives of people diagnosed 'schizophrenic' found that the most commonly endorsed causes were 'stress' and 'psychological traumas' with 68% of them believing that schizophrenia is caused entirely by psychosocial factors.[21] The finding is consistent across a range of cultures. Relatives in Turkey cited stressful events (50%) and family conflicts (40%) more often than biological/genetic factors (23%).[22] Similarly, 55% of Indian relatives cited social stressors, whereas only 5% cited heredity and 14% brain disorder.[23]

Further evidence of relatives' rejection of biogenetic beliefs comes from research into 'psycho-education' programmes specifically designed to teach them the illness model. One study assessed relatives' retention of 'knowledge' about the 'illness' and found 'absolutely no change in the amount of knowledge between pretests and posttests'.[24] Another found that before psycho-education only 11% of relatives believed the problems were caused by a 'disordered brain' and only 32% believed this after the training. Belief in 'genetic inheritance' increased from 11% to 15%. Only 3% of the patients adopted an illness model before or after the programme.[25]

Prejudice: Another major cause of mental health problems

The ill-informed and frequently unpleasant stereotypes that some people hold about people with mental health problems cannot be said to be an actual cause of the problems in the first place. Nevertheless, prejudice is a huge factor in preventing people from recovering from their difficulties. This is especially true if you internalise the negative attitudes and really start believing that you are inferior, useless, damaged or even dangerous etc. In Chapter 7 we will see that the cognitive model argues that what we tell ourselves about ourselves is a major cause of things like depression. If we are faced with negative attitudes from some members of the public (and some mental health staff) it can be even harder to start replacing our pre-existing negative thoughts with more positive ones. This is a serious issue. Prejudice against people with mental health problems is not just a set of privately held attitudes. Research has found that the prejudice is often acted upon, in terms of blatant discrimination in, for instance, employment and housing. The stereotypes for people deemed to be 'schizophrenic' are the worst of all, with dangerousness and unpredictability at the core of a very toxic set of beliefs.

   Although not directly relevant to our thinking about the causes of mental health problems, it is interesting to note how psychiatry has responded to all this prejudice and discrimination. Most 'destigmatisation' programmes around the world, usually funded by drug companies, have adopted the approach of trying to 'educate' us that we are wrong to believe that our problems are caused by events in our lives, and to persuade us instead that we have an 'illness' caused by some kind of biochemical imbalance. This 'mental illness is an illness like any other' approach to reducing prejudice is based on the well-intentioned idea that if a person is ill they cannot be held responsible for their actions and therefore cannot be blamed. Well-intentioned, but wrong.

All the research investigating the relationship between what we believe about causes and how prejudiced we are goes in the opposite direction. Studies show that the more we believe in biogenetic, illness-type causes, the more prejudiced and frightened we are of 'mental patients'.[26,27,28] Here is just one example. A research student of John's made a video (not unlike those used in professional training courses) of a young man (an actor) talking about hearing voices and believing that everyone was out to get him, followed by a doctor giving an explanation of the causes of these 'symptoms'. He showed the video to three groups of young people, but there was a different explanation given by the doctor at the end for each of the groups. The first group was told these were symptoms of the brain disease 'schizophrenia', the second were told the symptoms were caused by a combination of biological and social factors, and the third were told the voices and paranoia were reactions to trauma in the person's life. Attitudes were measured before and after the videos. In the first group (brain disease, schizophrenia) perceptions of 'dangerousness' and 'unpredictability' significantly increased. For the other two groups these negative attitudes decreased.[29] It doesn't help, it seems, to persuade us that the brains and genes of people who are struggling to cope are somehow very different from those of the rest of us. All the research from other fields about how to combat prejudice tells us that you have to emphasise similarities not differences. And when your strategy to reduce the prejudice and stigma includes telling people that the differences are due to unchangeable brain abnormalities of defective genes, then it is hardly surprising that this approach actually makes it worse.

Biological psychiatrists have been trying for more than half a century to get us to think like them. In 1961 the US's Joint Commission on Mental Illness and Health concluded:

> The principle of sameness as applied to the mentally sick versus the physically sick has become a cardinal tenet of mental health education ... Psychiatry has tried diligently to make society see the mentally ill in its way and has railed at the public's antipathy or indifference.[30]

We have known for a decade or two that this approach increases rather than decreases prejudice. It makes sense, of course, that the drug companies would disregard this and continue to cough up millions for 'destigmatisation' campaigns that continue to push the illness model. But it seems unforgiveable that some mental health professionals should go along with it. It is certainly unscientific.

What the public believes is, of course, just a set of beliefs, not 'scientific fact'. But the same is true of the tiny numbers of people – mostly biological psychiatrists and drug company employees – who believe the opposite. We shall see in the next chapter whether the research tends to support the ideas of the majority or the ideas of the minority.

What does seem to be a fact is that despite a concerted attempt, spanning 60 years or so and involving huge amounts of money, to persuade us that we are wrong to focus on the obvious, social causes of our problems, the ones we might be able to do something about, we remain, all over the world, unconvinced.

Chapter 6
Are the public right? What the research says about the causes of mental health problems

In the previous chapter we looked at the research surveying the views of non-professionals, including patients and family members. We saw survey respondents in different countries consistently identify the social causes of mental health problems, including:

in the UK
- life events, family problems and economic hardship
- social stressors and family conflicts – e.g., being mercilessly persecuted by family and friends
- having come from backgrounds that promote stress
- unusual or traumatic experiences
- social, economic, and family pressures

in Australia
- day-to-day-problems such as stress, family arguments, difficulties at work or financial difficulties
- the recent death of a close friend or relative
- traumatic events
- problems from childhood such as being badly treated or abused, losing one or both parents when young or coming from a broken home

in Ireland
- stressful life events
- childhood problems such as lack of adequate parental love

in Germany
- acute stress in the form of life events
- chronic stress in partnership and family

in the USA
- the way the person was raised
- stressful circumstances

The public seem to recognise two general groups of social causes: past and present. The causes in the past tend to focus, unsurprisingly, on childhood. The causes in the present are ongoing stresses of various sorts. Some specific types of causes, some of which span past and present, childhood and adulthood, are: poverty, trauma/abuse/ violence, neglect, loss and general day-to-day stress.

Does research support these widely held public beliefs? The research summarised next focuses largely, but not only, on the more extreme mental health problems like psychosis and 'schizophrenia'. This is mainly because if we can demonstrate that something as supposedly biological as 'schizophrenia' is actually largely caused by social factors, then it should not be surprising that things like depression and anxiety are also primarily caused by things that happen in our lives. We shall pay more attention to depression in Chapter 8.

It should be stressed from the outset that it is usually a combination of the factors discussed here, rather than any one of them in isolation, that tend to tip people into extremely distressing experiences likely to be diagnosed as 'psychosis'. Poverty by itself, for example rarely causes mental health problems, but in combination with childhood neglect for example (the chances of which are greater if you grow up in a poor family), your chances of becoming extremely depressed are relatively high compared to someone who grew up in a safe, nurturing, relatively well-off family. Furthermore, the richer you are, the more resources, professional or otherwise, you have at your disposal to help you through emotionally difficult times – an old joke says rich people holiday in the Bahamas while the rest of us take our 'breaks' in the loony bin.

Poverty

Mental hospitals have been filled predominantly with poor people throughout history. In 17th-century France, for example, the people confined in the Hôpital Général were 'the poor of Paris' (see also Chapter 2). The first of many studies in the 20th century, in 1939, found that the deprived central areas of Chicago had higher psychiatric admission rates than the wealthier suburbs. Contrary to the notion that milder mental health problems, but not schizophrenia, are socially caused, the difference was particularly high for 'schizophrenia'. People in the poorest areas of Chicago were seven times more likely to be diagnosed schizophrenic than those in the richest parts. This relationship between poverty and a diagnosis of schizophrenia was quickly replicated in nine other cities throughout the USA.[1] During the 1950s the same relationship was found in Bristol, Liverpool and London, as well as in Norway.[2]

A famous USA study[3] found that the poorest class (V: 'unskilled, manual') was three times more likely than the wealthiest two classes (I & II: 'business, professional and managerial') to be treated for psychiatric problems in general.

The diagnosis having the strongest relationship with class was schizophrenia. The poorest people were eight times more likely to be diagnosed as schizophrenic than the wealthiest.

By 1976 a review concluded:

> There have been more than 50 studies of the relationship between social class and rates of schizophrenia. Almost without exception, these studies have shown that schizophrenia occurs most frequently at the lowest social class levels of urban society. The evidence comes from research in Canada, Denmark, Finland, Great Britain, Norway, Sweden, Taiwan, and the United States – an unusually large number of countries and cultures for establishing the generality of any relationship in social science.[4]

Next, a New York study of first admissions found that Class V were 12 times more likely to be hospitalised than Class I, whilst a Tennessee study of 10,000 first admissions confirmed that schizophrenia was the diagnosis most strongly related to socio-economic status. The relationship between schizophrenia and poverty was described as 'one of the most consistent findings in the field of psychiatric epidemiology'.[5]

Since 1980, the relationship between poverty and being admitted to a psychiatric hospital has been confirmed, again, in Bristol, London, Nottingham, Wales, Finland, New Zealand, Canada, and Nigeria.[6] More often than not the strongest relationship between class and psychiatric admission is for 'schizophrenia'.

A British study found that deprived children are four times more likely to develop 'non-schizophrenic psychotic illness' but eight times more likely to grow up to be 'schizophrenic' than non-deprived children.[7] Even among children with no family history of psychosis, the deprived children were seven times more likely to develop schizophrenia, questioning the whole idea of a genetic predisposition.

Whilst poverty is particularly predictive of schizo-phrenia,[8] it is also predictive of a host of other mental health problems, including depression, generalised anxiety disorders, phobias, panic disorder, alcohol abuse, drug abuse, erectile dysfunction, and childhood 'disorders' such as 'conduct disorder'. For example, a 2007 study covering 14 USA states found that admission to hospital for depression was significantly predicted by both poverty and unemployment.[9] A 2008 British study that has followed nearly 10,000 people since their birth in 1958 found that those who were poor at age 7 were significantly more likely to have, at age 45, generalised anxiety disorder, depressive episodes, phobias and panic disorder.[10]

It must also be noted that there is very convincing evidence that *relative* poverty is a stronger predictor than poverty per se. In their book, *The Spirit Level* (and on www.equalitytrust.org.uk), British epidemiologists Richard Wilkinson and Kate Pickett report multiple studies demonstrating a far stronger relationship between relative poverty and a range of social, health and mental health outcomes than between poverty per se and the same outcomes.[11] They first note that in many countries rates of mental illness and levels of inequality have both increased significantly in recent decades. They then report a strong relationship between degree of income inequality and rates of people meeting diagnostic criteria for mental illness over a 12-month period, across 12 countries (see Figure 1). Similar findings are reported for other outcomes, including level of use of illegal drugs (Figure 2). In another recent book, psychologist and journalist Oliver James coined the term 'Affluenza' to describe and explain this phenomenon.[12]

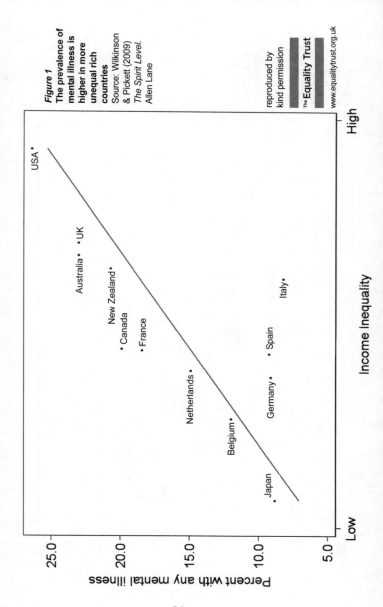

Figure 1
The prevalence of mental illness is higher in more unequal rich countries
Source: Wilkinson & Pickett (2009) *The Spirit Level.* Allen Lane

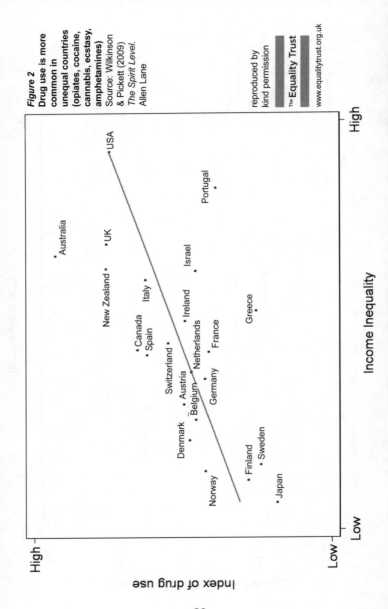

Figure 2
Drug use is more common in unequal countries (opiates, cocaine, cannabis, ecstasy, amphetamines)
Source: Wilkinson & Pickett (2009) *The Spirit Level.* Allen Lane

82

Urbanicity

Growing up or living in large cites is also a factor in a wide range of mental health problems, including depression and substance abuse. Again, the relationship is even stronger for schizophrenia than for other diagnoses.[13] Not only is being diagnosed 'schizophrenic' associated with living in urban areas, but the greater the numbers of years lived in urban areas *prior to diagnosis*, the greater the risk of being diagnosed 'schizophrenic' later in life.[14]

Two further studies confirm the influence of psychosocial factors in the absence of the supposed genetic predisposition to 'schizophrenia'. The relationship between urban living and schizophrenia remains after controlling for family history of psychiatric disorder in general, or of schizophrenia specifically. The 'attributable risk' from urban birth was four times greater than that from having a mother with 'schizophrenia'.[15]

Ethnicity

The relationship between ethnicity and mental health problems is complex and hotly debated. We include brief mention of it under 'poverty' to indicate that the demonstrated relationship between a range of mental health problems and belonging to an indigenous group or an 'ethnic minority' has little to do with the race or culture itself and everything to do with the social circumstances in which many members of such groups are forced to live, including discrimination and poverty.

Ethnicity is a powerful predictor of a diagnosis of schizophrenia. This has been demonstrated in Australia, Belgium, Denmark, Germany, Greenland, the Netherlands, New Zealand, Israel, Sweden, the UK and the USA.[16] In the

UK, for example, the incidence rates for schizophrenia are 3.6 times higher among all ethnic minority groups combined than among whites. Afro-Caribbeans have been found to be 9 to 12 times more likely to be diagnosed schizophrenic than white people.[17] Although racist misdiagnoses are part of the explanation, the factors that link ethnicity to 'schizophrenia' are poverty, unemployment, discrimination, and social isolation. Janssen at al. recorded experiences of discrimination in 4,067 Dutch people.[18] Those who had reported discrimination in two or more domains (skin colour/ ethnicity, gender, age etc.) were three times more likely to be experiencing psychotic hallucinations than those who had reported no discrimination, and five times more likely to be experiencing psychotic delusions. A study of over 10,000 Swedes, looking at a range of problems including depression, concluded that 'the association between immigrant status and mental illness appears above all to be an effect of a higher prevalence of social and economic disadvantage.[19]

Trauma

The public, as we have seen, have no difficulty grasping that mental health problems, by and large, are caused by bad things happening to us. Even the American Psychiatric Association has included 'post-traumatic stress disorder' (PTSD) in the DSM – see Chapter 4. Interestingly, this diagnosis (the only one of the hundreds in the DSM to acknowledge the social cause of a problem in its name), did not become an official diagnosis (in 1968) because of the recognition of the effects of violence against children and women, but because of the thousands of men returning to the USA in a traumatised state from the Vietnam war.

Traumatic events, however, contribute to a much wider range of mental health problems than PTSD, including the most common ones like depression and anxiety disorders. There is now a significant, wide-ranging and unignorable body of research documenting that the public are right when they think that things like child abuse, rape and violent assaults in adulthood, war traumas and so on are extremely powerful factors involved in a vast array of mental health problems. Only tiny fractions of this research can be summarised here, as examples.

It is true, of course, that not everyone exposed to abuse or violence ends up with terrifying, disabling experiences and a serious mental health diagnosis. Research and common sense tell us that the best indicators of which abused/assaulted people end up in a bad state are:

- if the abuse occurs early in life
- if there are multiple incidents or types of abuse
- if it is inflicted by a loved one on whom we are dependent
- in the case of child abuse, whether we managed to tell someone soon afterwards and were believed and supported or whether we were told to keep it a secret and internalized the experience

Child abuse

A recent review of 59 studies of the most severely disturbed 'psychiatric patients' found that 64% of the women and 55% of the men had been physically or sexually abused as children.[20] Most of the physical abuse was inflicted by family members. For more than half of the sexually abused females and about a quarter of the sexually abused males, the abuser was a family member (incest).[21]

Psychiatric patients subjected to childhood sexual or physical abuse have earlier first admissions to hospital, longer and more frequent hospitalisations, spend longer in seclusion, receive more medication, are more likely to self-mutilate, and have higher global symptom severity.[22,23]

Psychiatric patients who were abused as children are also far more likely to try to kill themselves. Two New Zealand studies, one general population study and one of a clinical sample, illustrate the strength of the relationship between child abuse and suicidality. A survey of over 2,000 women found that those who had been sexually abused as children were 19 times more likely to have tried to kill themselves (and seven times more likely to have been admitted to a psychiatric hospital). Those who had been physically abused were five times more likely to have tried to commit suicide.[24] A study of 200 adult psychiatric outpatients found that child abuse (on average about 20 years earlier) was a better predictor of current suicidality than a current diagnosis of depression.[25]

Child abuse is now known to have a significant causal role in most mental health problems, including depression, anxiety disorders, PTSD, eating disorders, sexual difficulties, substance abuse, personality disorders, and dissociative disorders.

The relationship between child abuse and psychosis or schizophrenia, John's main research area, is still seen by some biological psychiatrists as rather controversial. But his 2008 review of the research literature found that ten of the last eleven large-scale studies found convincing evidence of the relationship.[26]

Child neglect and emotional abuse
More subtle, ongoing childhood circumstances can be just as damaging to our long-term mental health as more blatant events like being sexually molested or repeatedly beaten. The absence of love ('emotional neglect'), or of the basics of

life ('physical neglect'), or being repeatedly told you are 'rubbish' or 'useless' ('emotional abuse') have all, unsurprisingly, also been linked to a whole range of mental health problems later in life.

The survey of 2,000 New Zealand women found that those who had been emotionally abused were three times more likely to be depressed or to have sexual problems, four times more likely to have an eating disorder, five times more likely to have had a psychiatric admission and twelve times more likely to have tried to commit suicide. Studies elsewhere around the world produce similar results. The 2008 review mentioned above found, in six studies of adults diagnosed 'schizophrenic', the following average rates: emotional neglect – 51%, physical neglect – 41%, and emotional abuse – 47%.

Bullying
Being repeatedly picked on or beaten up at school (sometimes, made worse these days by the added humiliation of having the incidents broadcast on the Internet) can obviously lower our self-esteem, lead to depression, destroy our trust in other people in general, and, at its extreme, lead (understandably) to paranoia. For example, people in England who were bullied as children or adolescents have been found to be four times more likely to be diagnosed as psychotic later in life.[27]

Rape and violence in adulthood
Being raped or physically assaulted are most obviously connected to PTSD. The three major 'symptom' groups of PTSD are heightened vigilance, re-experiencing symptoms (flashbacks, dreams etc.), and avoidance (of certain social situations and of feelings – 'numbing'). These 'symptoms' become perfectly understandable once the trauma (rape,

assault etc.) is known about. Again however, our diagnostic symptom – designed to put people into boxes – often masks the fact that interpersonal violence can also lead to a whole range of other difficulties including depression, phobias, dissociative disorders and, yet again, psychosis and schizophrenia.

Most psychiatric patients suffer serious assaults as adults. It is difficult, of course, to determine which comes first, the violence or the unusual behaviour which might have provoked the powerful negative stereotypes about mad people and then led to the violence. It is also true that when severely disturbed, we can be particularly vulnerable to predators and others inclined to violence.[28] One study found that in the year prior to psychiatric hospitalisation, 63% suffered violence by partners and 46% of those living at home were assaulted by family members. Sexual assaults as adults are experienced by the majority of female patients and about a quarter of male patients.[29]

War trauma

Seeing people killed, while your own life is simultaneously at risk, can lead not only to PTSD, but a range of other severe difficulties. Again, this includes psychosis, which has been linked in research studies not just to combat veterans but also prisoners of war, war rape victims, refugees from the Pol Pot regime and from war in Somalia, people exposed to bombings, shootings, and 'punishment' beatings in Northern Ireland, and Holocaust survivors.[30,31,32]

Loss

Losing a loved one can, of course, fall into the category of 'trauma'. We have given it its own section, however, because loss, in its various forms, is such a huge cause of mental health problems and because, like child abuse, it sometimes doesn't receive the attention it deserves from those mental health professionals who see our problems as biologically based 'illnesses'.

Like poverty, loss by itself does not necessarily lead to mental health problems. The sadness we feel when mourning the death of a loved one is *not* a mental health problem (although some doctors are happy to 'treat' it as such by prescribing antidepressants or tranquillisers practically on request). As discussed earlier, a combination of factors is usually required before we get into serious emotional difficulties. Three of the more obvious factors that can influence whether we come through a period of mourning in reasonably good shape after a loss are: (i) whether we have recently experienced other significant losses; (ii) how much support and understanding we get while mourning; and (iii) how close we were to the loved one we lost.

A fourth exacerbating factor is being told by a professional that your sadness is a sign of some kind of mental illness, such as a 'depressive disorder'. This can both invalidate your feelings *and* make you worry that there is something seriously and irreversibly wrong with you for feeling so down. This can interfere with the natural grieving process and, ironically, help lock you into a longer period of depression than if you had just been left with your normal social supports for time to do its healing thing.

Given the increasing medicalisation of everything in life, mental health professionals who confuse grieving with 'mental illness' are not helped by brain researchers, often funded by the drug companies, who produce studies showing, unsurprisingly, that when we are feeling sad or depressed our brains operate differently. This leads the researchers, and some mental health practitioners, to conclude that it is the brain that has caused the depression. We believe it is the other way round, i.e., that the brain is reacting to, not causing, the depressing event, loss or otherwise. This is, after all, what the brain is supposed to do. It is the organ in our body that reacts and adjusts to the environment, helping us adapt to a changing world. If it did not operate differently in circumstances such as bereavement and loss, it would be a cause for concern.

It is also true, however, that the longer the brain stays in its depressed state the harder it can be for it to return to its non-depressed state, hence the temptation to try to kick-start it back to 'normality' with chemicals or electric shocks. The DSM approach (see Chapter 4) to the challenge of deciding when, after the death of a loved one, our sadness and lack of motivation to do everyday things is a natural grieving process and when it is a mental disorder is interesting. The DSM states that for the first 60 days it is natural but on the 61st day it becomes a 'major depressive episode'. The psychiatrists involved in drawing this line have, at least, acknowledged that sadness after loss is normal – but only up to a point. Where would you draw the line? Clearly if you are still feeling dreadful and unable to get on with your life five years after the death of your husband, wife, mother or father then that is a problem. What about three years? One year? There are individual differences (again, everyone is different) and cultural variations which sometimes lead to jokes suggesting that more than half an hour grieving for the stiff-upper-lipped English would be indicative of major depression while less than a twelve-month wake for the more emotionally expressive Irish would be problematic. We are not trying to make light of a difficult life event – simply trying to get across the futility of setting an arbitrary cut-off point at which mourning becomes a mental illness. We never tire of repeating that people are all different and some of those differences are determined by the culture and family we grew up in, because the medical model of mental illness and psychiatric diagnosis are determined to pathologise the naturally variable grieving process.

It is our life history before the loss (including how many other losses we have suffered), combined with the response of others around us, and the quality of our life outside the lost relationship (and, yes, our cultural norms) that determine how long we grieve – not whether or not we have a mental disorder, whether or not there is something wrong with our genes or the neurotransmitters in our brains.

Loss comes in many shapes and sizes – we are not only talking about death of someone close to us. We all lose friendships and romantic relationships and losses occur all the time in less personal areas of our lives. The loss of a job can be devastating financially and, if our self-esteem is highly determined by our work status, emotionally.

We guess that most readers will not have got through the year without suffering one or more of the following:

- the death of a loved one
- a miscarriage
- the break up of a marriage or life-partnership
- a son or daughter leaving home
- losing your job
- being robbed or burgled
- losing money on a bad investment
- your favoured political party losing an election

Perhaps, in a very good year, your biggest loss might be that your football team yet again fails to win the league. (It has happened to both of us every year for the past 40 years.)

Some losses are less obvious than others. One type of

loss that often goes unnoticed is the loss of our hopes. The continuous failure to realise any of our aspirations can be as chronically damaging as some of the more obvious, one-off losses discussed above. Some people, the relatively well-off for instance, have a better chance of having some of their dreams come true than others. A feeling of loss can also occur when we realise that we didn't get something that most others did get (or that we *persuade ourselves* most others got), or that we feel we should have had – we realise that our childhood circumstances represent a loss. A 'lost childhood' is a term familiar to us all. We usually mean that the child was not provided with the basics, physically or emotionally, or was subjected to things no child should have to endure. We mention these less tangible losses to draw readers' attention to the full range of losses that should be considered when trying to figure out where our 'problems' have come from.

Whilst it is folk wisdom that time heals, and whilst this may be true, it is also important to acknowledge that some losses, like the death of a son or daughter for instance, fall into a category of losses that may never be completely 'recovered' from. Some losses inevitably remain an important part of the rest of our lives, and should be. This does not mean there is something wrong with us, that we have a mental disorder. However, that, in turn does *not* mean that we don't sometimes need help from other people, relatives, friends and even occasionally, professionals (preferably someone who, like the public, understands that being depressed after a loss makes sense).

Before offering just one or two research studies demonstrating the obvious link between loss and mental health difficulties, we should touch on one more factor, namely, that two people experiencing a similar loss, let's say of a spouse, can react quite differently. We have already mentioned other personal determining factors, such as other recent losses and the reactions of those around us. Yet another factor is what we tell ourselves about the loss. If we decide it was our fault, partly or completely, for instance, we are more likely to be more depressed, and to stay depressed for longer. If, after losing a job, you believe it was because your boss is a fool or because the economic system is rubbish, you may well feel angry. But you will probably feel less depressed than if you tell yourself that you lost your job because you are incompetent or useless and therefore deserved to lose it.

What we tell ourselves is particularly important after the extremely distressing event of the suicide of someone we love. It is almost impossible, when that happens, not to dwell on what you might have done differently, to blame yourself in some way. Any anger at the person who committed suicide can get buried under endless self-recrimination. This is true for mental health professionals too. Some of them, especially those who work with the most distressed people, will experience suicides of people they have genuinely come to care about. If you try hard enough you will indeed find something you could have done, or not done, that *might* have made a difference.

The point is that whether or not we blame ourselves for the loss will play a part in how long it takes us to move on. We will return to this important cause of mental health problems – our thoughts and beliefs – when we look briefly at cognitive theory in the next chapter.

It might seem unnecessary to provide research evidence that folk wisdom and public opinion are right to assume that a serious loss, or multiple losses, can play a significant role in the development of mental health problems. But since current mental health treatment provision in practice is likely to pathologise grieving and prioritise medication over talking therapies we will mention just two of the many studies available. Again they focus on the type of problems that many psychiatrists believe are most biological and least social in origin – 'psychosis' and 'schizophrenia'.

A recent British study found that 390 people with a first episode of psychosis were twice as likely as a control group to have been separated for at least a year from one of their parents before age 16, three times more likely to have had one of their parents die, and twelve times more likely to have had their mother die.[33] These findings were after controlling for parental history of mental illness, yet again casting doubt on the genetic predisposition requirement for psychosis. As is the case for child abuse, the younger the child is when the loss occurs the greater the potential long-term consequences. Among people who had lost a parent in childhood those who were later diagnosed with 'schizophrenia' has lost the parent an average of two years earlier (at an average age of about six years old) than a control group. An Israeli study found that death of, or permanent separation from, a parent was only predictive of 'schizophrenia' if occurring in the first eight years of life.[34]

Day-to-day stress

The public is also right to identify, as major causes of mental health problems, things like: 'life events', 'family problems', 'social stressors', 'social, economic, and family pressures', 'day-to-day-problems such as stress, family arguments, difficulties at work or financial difficulties', 'stressful life events' 'acute stress in the form of life events', 'chronic stress in partnership and family' and 'stressful circumstances'. This seems so obvious that we will not waste space on research studies demonstrating that stress levels are related to just about every mental health problem in the

DSM. It seems some of us are more sensitive to stressors than others. While professionals and academics might quibble about whether this variation in sensitivity depends on our genes or our childhoods (we think the answer is both) we almost all agree that day-to-day stress is hugely important in determining who cracks up, or gives up, and who doesn't.

Conclusion

Of course there are other causes of mental health problems. And the causes are different for each one of us. They can even be different for us, as individuals, at different points in our lives, depending on what is happening around us. We have merely tried to identify some of the most common causes found by research studies. Academics, of course, have their own biases and tend to research what they think are causes in the first place. We probably miss other causes in the process. An example of this comes from the vitally important field of suicide research. Traditional, biologically oriented researchers investigate whether people who kill themselves have high rates of an illness called 'depression'. Researchers who find this rather meaningless and are more interested in *why* people get so depressed, tend to research things like child abuse. Both groups find their hypotheses confirmed! A few years ago one of John's research students wanted to address the issue of New Zealand's high youth suicide rate without any preconceptions or specific hypotheses. She decided to simply ask several hundred young New Zealanders (in the same age 18–24 age bracket which had the highest suicide rate) why *they* think the rate is so high. The most commonly cited cause of suicide was pressure to conform and perform, followed by financial worries, abuse and neglect, problems with alcohol or drugs, and boredom. Mental illness was cited by only 1%. Many people probably would not have thought of pressure to conform and perform, and would definitely never thought of boredom, as contributors.

Having discussed a rather long list of possible causes, the *what* in the 'causes' puzzle, we move on in the next chapter to discuss *how* these various factors lead to mental health problems.

To listen to a 2005 public debate at the Institute of Psychiatry in London at which John proposed the motion that 'Child abuse is a cause of schizophrenia', go to: http://www.iop.kcl.ac.uk/podcast/ ?id=208&type=item

Chapter 7
Psychological theories: *How* events operate on us to create problems

Do you think mental health problems come about largely because some people tell themselves negative things about themselves? Do you prefer to think about patterns of relationships we develop early in life and then repeat over and over again? Maybe you think that distress is an understandable, if extreme, coping reaction to distressing life events and that if health-promoting conditions prevail, we have the capacity to recover ourselves? Perhaps you like the idea that we learn unhelpful ways of behaving from having them reinforced in the past? Or do you value thinking about unconscious desires and conflicts? We all have our preferred ways of understanding ourselves and other people, although we may not all – like some psychologists – be bold enough to turn them into formal theories.

There are many psychological theories around about how human beings develop their patterns of behaving, thinking and feeling. These are called 'personality theories', 'developmental theories' or 'psychological models'. They try to explain both 'normal' and 'abnormal' ways of interacting with the world, or as Pete has previously written, '... the study of personality is the study of human psychological structure – how people are *put together*, how they *work* and ... how they *fall apart*.'[1]

Each of the many theories has different explanations of the causes of mental health problems and carries the ideas through to form the bases of different types of psychological treatments. So a psychodynamic/psychoanalytic therapist will follow the theory developed by Sigmund Freud and his followers, a humanistic person-centred therapist will base their ideas and practice on the work of Carl Rogers, whilst a cognitive therapist will see value in and follow the theory and techniques suggested by the work of people like Aaron Beck.

Understanding a little about the six theories summarised here may help you think through how psychological problems start and develop into life-affecting distress. It may also help you understand how therapy can help clients figure out what is currently getting in the way of overcoming (or accepting) them. This knowledge may also help you understand what psychologists, counsellors or psychotherapists think and what they are trying to do to help their patients or clients. However, we would always suggest that a good mental health professional should explain their theory or model to their clients at the outset. If they don't – clients should ask them!

You will already lean towards certain explanations according to your family culture, religious beliefs, education and experiences in life – including, most importantly, your experiences of mental distress. The ideas and language we use when thinking and talking about psychological distress are a clue to how we might lean towards different theories. We will see as we go along how, over the years, the language of psychological theories has crept into our everyday thinking. We suggest here that, after considering all the theories summarised, you take what makes sense to you and, again, like Paul Simon, 'disregard the rest'.

Psychoanalysis

Before we get into introducing the ideas of Sigmund Freud, we need to explain something about the current use of terminology. 'Psychoanalysis' usually refers to a rather strict belief in the original teachings of Sigmund Freud – who, understandably, is revered by some in the mental health world. 'Psychodynamic' is a broader term which includes psychoanalysis and all the many ideas that have built upon, and branched out from, Freud's original theories. We should also point out that over time Freud, and indeed all major players in psychological theory, revised and developed their own ideas, which were further revised and developed by their students and followers later.

Psychodynamic theories can be quite complicated. So if you try reading some of these folk and you don't get it, don't think you need to keep at it till it sinks in – maybe it's just not for you. Move on until you find something that makes sense. Psychodynamic (and humanistic) thinkers include factors that are hard to measure – in the case of psychodynamic theories, things like the unconscious, dreams and so on. They are often criticised by more hard-nosed psychologists for not being 'scientific'. Maybe you have your own thoughts on how scientific psychology should be. One problem is that there is more than one view about what exactly constitutes science, but unfortunately we don't have the space to look at that issue at all, let alone in any detail. We'll confine ourselves to the content of the theories and leave you to make your own mind up.

Human development
Freud thought that human adult personality is the result of a few fundamental elements of humanness developed into a unique person by early experiences. He reasoned that all

humans go through the same set of life experiences as they develop into adults. Namely, all have to be weaned onto solid food, all have to learn to control their bowels, all have to develop their sexuality and all have to become capable of separate existence from their parents. These milestones of human development are achieved in all cultures, but in each culture (including, of course, each family) by slightly different means. Each culture and each family within that culture has different rituals and practices to achieve these transitions.

Without going into detail, suffice it to say that Freud and his followers thought that how these landmark events are handled by each family leads to differences between us in terms of how we react to the world. For example, the sort of things that we get anxious about, the ways we seek comfort and how much we want to control our surroundings are all thought to be due to the way these important, essential life stages were conducted, from overly controlling to overly permissive parenting.

As we proceed through these stages of development our essential humanness is unfolding. The interaction between the two (developmental transitions and unfolding essential humanness) weaves our personality into three parts. These three parts are:

Id This is the part of the personality that we are born with. Freud described the id as a seething cauldron of instincts and desires which seek gratification at all costs. Id processes are unconscious. Not only are we not aware of them, but they are so primitive and survival oriented they are almost dangerous and chaotic and are ultimately pleasure- and comfort-seeking. The id has no values, morals or concept of right and wrong. Its workings are most clearly seen in the behaviour of a new-born baby. Freud called the inborn energy of the id the life energy or *libido* and he believed that it was largely sexual in nature.

Super-ego This is the conscience, the internalised parent part of the personality. Freud believed that the super-ego formed when the child identifies with the same-sex parent, changing 'You mustn't do this' to 'I mustn't do this' so internalising rules, morals, notions of right and wrong, sex roles, etc. The development of the super-ego is basically a learning process. The strength of the super-ego is accounted for by the fact that it develops at a very early age (around five years old) when young children are very vulnerable and impressionable.

Ego The ego develops through childhood, first as a mediator between the chaotic id and the outside world. The ego works out the consequences of behaviour aimed at satisfying the id and applies the brakes to the id impulses based on reality. Later the ego has to appease the demands of the super-ego, so its task becomes a delicate balancing act. The ego is only fully developed at maturity. A properly adjusted adult is governed by the ego, balancing the 'I want it now!' demands of the id against the 'You mustn't do this you naughty boy!' admonishments of the super-ego.

Freud proposed that there were three domains of mental life: the *conscious* domain, the *pre-conscious* domain and the *unconscious* domain. We might picture these domains stacked on top of each other with the unconscious at the bottom; inaccessible, hidden and unknown. The pre-conscious is in the middle acting as a half-way house and the conscious on top; known, available and present as the mediator of everyday living.

The unconscious is the domain of the taboo id impulses which are the source of the very life of the organism, being concerned with survival, sex, comfort, and bodily functions. These impulses must be kept hidden from our awareness, confined to the unconscious domain, denied admission to the conscious in their raw, rather offensive, animalistic form. It is by keeping these impulses 'in their proper place' that a healthy dynamic equilibrium is maintained by the ego. However, there is a problem. As well as being taboo, the id energy is also life-giving and life-sustaining; it is the source of our creative energy and we need these impulses to live a fulfilling life.

The ego defends the conscious mind against raw id impulses by creating a barrier thorough which they can only gain admission by various roundabout ways, becoming acceptable in the process. This re-routing takes the form of what are called *ego defences* or *defence mechanisms*. Since id energy *must* gain expression somehow we are all using defence mechanisms all of the time.

Ego defences can be successful: allowing expression of the forbidden impulse in a way that gives the id satisfaction; or unsuccessful: simply preventing expression and causing the impulse to re-present itself over and over again, each time demanding satisfaction. Unsuccessful ego-defence leaves undischarged energy in the system which must go somewhere and so is eventually expressed as anxiety. Defence mechanisms are not necessarily pathological; they serve, for all of us, the invaluable function of keeping undesirable drives, feelings and memories out of awareness. Without defence mechanisms we would be completely unable to get on with our day-to-day lives. Yet Freud believed that some were healthier than others.

Successful ego-defence is called *sublimation* and is achieved by deflecting the impulse into an acceptable activity, so:

- the desire to handle faeces becomes an interest in pottery
- the impulse to be aggressive is satisfied by playing competitive sport

There are lots of less successful ego defences – including, for example:

Repression is the process of keeping taboo impulses and any related ideas out of consciousness – so that we are completely unaware of them. Recently, the idea of repression has been applied to memories of childhood abuse. The recovery of such memories is a matter of hot debate amongst psychologists.

Reaction-formation is the formation of feelings in the conscious that are the opposite of the unconscious id impulses. Examples are love becoming hate (most teenagers will understand this!), whilst over-moralising and disgust are reactions against sexuality.

Projection is the attribution of our own taboo impulses to others. So 'I hate him' becomes 'he hates me'. Combined with reaction-formation we can see how a chain of events develops; 'I love him' becomes 'I hate him' (via reaction-formation) which in turn becomes 'He hates me' (via projection). Since the original taboo impulses are unconscious and therefore not known to us, this chain of events is out of our awareness and the first we know is that we get a strong notion that a new acquaintance dislikes us from the off. So, a common form of projection is when self-hatred (which is unacceptable) is projected onto the other person as 'You don't like me,' or, 'You hate me!'

Turning against self might seem to be an idea in conflict with projection, but it is yet another way of denying an unacceptable impulse. This time if I have aggressive feelings towards someone I love (an unacceptable impulse) I can turn them back upon myself. This leads to self-doubt, self-loathing and in extreme cases, self-harm and suicide.

Dreams

You can't really talk about psychoanalysis without mentioning dreams. Freud called them 'the royal road to the unconscious'. While the usually vigilant ego is taking a break, the id is free to run rampant. Along with 'Freudian slips' (e.g., 'Hello. I don't believe we've been properly seduced') dreams can help us discover our deeper desires and fears, however surprising or unflattering they may be. If you want to use your own dreams to help you understand yourself do not buy a dream dictionary that tells you, for instance, that all trains represent penises and all tunnels, vaginas. Freud was very clear that we develop our own symbols. So, instead, buy a notebook, and (when you can catch your dreams in the morning – which is the hard part because the ego wakes up pretty fast and puts the lid back on) jot down as much as you can remember. After a few weeks have a read through and see what comes to you. And remember that not all dreams are deep and meaningful. Some are just a mindless repeating of the boring events of the day before!

Freud's disciples

Freud's ideas were spread by his students and followers to the extent that now hundreds of thousands of people all over the world practise what Freud preached. The better known of them are those that have dissented to some extent and established their own variations – we offer just a few of examples here. Carl Jung was one of the first to break ranks with his emphasis on the spiritual world, his belief in a *collective* unconscious, shared by all of us, and his ideas about our all being made up of opposite and competing parts like the archetypal female – Jung called it the 'anima' – and male, or 'animus' in us all. Frieda Fromm-Reichman and Harry Stack Sullivan developed Freud's understanding of psychosis in terms of what had happened to people and how that led them to distort the world.

Sándor Ferenczi seemed destined to become Freud's chosen successor until he insisted that Freud had been correct, early in his career, to point out that most of his female patients had been sexually abused as children. Freud had soon retracted his original belief that many of his clients had been sexually abused and replaced it with the idea that children fantasise about having sex with their parents. More recently, Jeffrey Masson was one psychoanalyst who didn't think it was a good idea to base a whole school of thought on the idea that if someone tells you they were abused as a child you should assume it was just a fantasy. He discovered, in Freud's unpublished letters, evidence that Freud never really stopped believing in sexual abuse as a primary cause of mental health problems and that he had been pressured into retracting his claim by pressure from his colleagues. His account of all this is in his book *Assault on Truth* (1984).[2]

We have no way of knowing whether a psychodynamic approach – or the other theories that follow – will be of any use to you in your thinking about the causes of your difficulties in life. We do know that some of the basic ideas of psychoanalytic theory make sense to and are accepted by millions of people around the world, with many of his basic ideas – like dream interpretation and 'Freudian slips' having become part of popular culture. Others find some psychoanalytic ideas hard to grasp and therefore rather irritating or even nonsensical. Perhaps start with a brief introductory text.[3]

Attachment theory

British psychiatrist John Bowlby was originally a psychoanalyst, but became interested in Konrad Lorenz's famous research into how young chicks, and other animals, become 'imprinted' on or attached to – and follow around – the first available adult (of any species, or indeed an inanimate object if it is in the right place at the right time). Bowlby's seminal work *Attachment and Loss* [4] – in which he presented the findings from his research for the World Health Organisation on homeless and orphaned children in post-war Europe – is still available and is the basis for modern-day attachment theory, and his book *Child Care and the Growth of Love*[5] influenced the provision of care for orphaned children throughout the developed world. His work is still instructive reading for anyone interested in the causes of mental health problems. Early separation from parents was a major problem in Britain during Word War II because of the deaths of so many men in active service, and the deaths of whole families due to bombing, and also the prolonged separation due to evacuation of children from the cities.

Bowlby's attachment theory argues that a baby's first relationship with an adult (usually the mum) is hugely important in how we relate to others as adults. He argued that the quality of that first relationship largely determines how we relate to other people when we are grown ups. At a very young age we develop 'internal models' of what we expect relationships to be like.

American researcher Mary Ainsworth used Bowlby's theory in her 'Strange Situation' experiment. She observed how toddlers react when their mum leaves a room, and also when she returns. She identified three 'attachment styles'. The first (shown by about 70% of the children) she called secure attachment. These children were a little upset when mum left but greeted her when she came back and were easily comforted. About 20% the children, with 'avoidant attachment', took little notice when mum left and avoided her when she returned. The third group (about 10%) had considerable difficulty separating from mum and when she came back alternated between wanting to be picked up and squirming to be put down. Ainsworth called this 'ambivalent attachment'.

Later research shows that these attachment styles, learned very early in life, do indeed influence our relationships as adults.[6] Unsurprisingly, those of us with a secure attachment style tend to find it fairly easy to make friends and to trust them. Those of us who learned an avoidant style find it difficult to depend on, and trust others, and often keep a safe distance that others sometimes find difficult. And if you picked up an ambivalent attachment style when little you may want to have a very close (almost merged) relationship with someone but spend a lot of time worrying about whether they love you as much as you love them and that they will leave you. This, understandably, tends to scare other people away.

More recent work on attachment styles is considered by some to apply to all approaches, in the sense that it is taken to be presenting 'universal truths' about the effects of impaired attachment. In particular, the work of psychodynamic psychologist Peter Fonagy, linking adult mental health to attachment styles whilst embracing neuropsychology, has captured the imagination of a number of psychotherapists and counsellors.[7] He goes into great detail about types of attachment, saying that stable adult mental health requires the attachment figure (usually the mother) to provide a relationship with is both contained (safe) and regulated. If the parent is themselves beset by problems, ranging from drug dependency through to poverty, their ability to provide the right sort of attachment relationship is compromised.

Be careful not to put yourself, or your parents or carers too rigidly in one of these apparent categories – these categories are not 'boxes', they are dimensions along which individuals fall at different points. It remains the case, though, that ideas about particular styles of attachment can sometimes be useful in trying to understand where a person's current difficulties started. Just remember, if you conclude that your parents or early caregivers did not help you develop a secure attachment style, that they had childhoods, and parents, too!

Learning theories

Learning theories are not concerned with early relationships with our mums or our dreams or unconscious fears and desires. Learning theories were at the centre of the emerging field of behaviourism in the early 20th century. The founders of behaviourism were, in their determination to make psychology scientific, only interested in things that could be reliably measured. The behavioural approaches, more than any other theory hitherto, used academic psychology as its starting point. Much of modern psychology owes a great deal to the work of early behaviourists. Behaviourism grew to all but dominate American psychology by the middle of the century. J.B. Watson and B.F. Skinner, working separately and on different learning processes, founded the movement which Skinner hoped would set humans free from the shackles of their existence by developing a technology of change and making it available to everyone – science to set everyone free.

The basic principles of behaviourism are:

• Apparently complex behaviour is a collection of more simple elements which can be understood in terms of basic learning principles.

• Whatever has been learned can be unlearned and modified through the application of learning principles. Careful unravelling the 'what has been learned' and 'how it was learned' is the key to understanding learning that has been unhelpful or led to distressing outcomes or symptoms. Once understood, it can be unlearned and more positive behaviour learned in its place.

There are two ways in which a new pattern of behaviour can be acquired – two types of learning. They are called classical conditioning and operant or instrumental conditioning.

Classical conditioning

Classical conditioning is a type of stimulus–response relationship where a stimulus becomes associated with a reflex response. Ivan Pavlov, a Russian physiologist studying the salivary reflex, stumbled on the procedure about 100 years ago. He noticed that if a dog was fed from the same bowl by the same lab technician repeatedly, the dog would start to salivate at the sight of the bowl alone and even at the sight of the lab technician. Note that salivation is a reflex that happens in anticipation of food to prepare for the digestion of food. Thousands of experiments followed, using the same principle. This principle, that a (previously) 'neutral' stimulus (the sight of the lab technician) can produce a 'conditioned response' (salivation) through its association with a stimulus (food) that automatically produces the same response, has provided a useful model to help us understand, for example, phobias.

John B. Watson, with his colleague Rosalie Rayner, conducted a famous experiment with an infant called Albert (the study became known as the 'Little Albert' experiment) in which they paired (presented together) a white rat (to which Albert had previously been attracted) and the loud noise of metal bar being struck by a hammer behind the child's head. Albert was frightened by the noise and began to associate the noise with the presence of the white rat. After a few pairings, Albert cried every time the rat was brought near him. This demonstrated that a fear reflex could be learned and associated with a neutral object – one way we could become fearful of 'neutral' objects, animals or situations.

Several classical conditioning experiments demonstrated the important idea of 'generalisation' whereby we can become fearful of things because they are similar to the stimulus we have become frightened of. Soldiers returning from active duty often find that they are panicked by any loud noise that is similar to their frightening battlefield experiences. Similarly people who have been abused as kids often feel fearful in the presence of someone who resembles the abuser. If other people don't know about our life histories we can look pretty mad if we 'overreact' (have a 'conditioned emotional reaction') to a car backfiring or to a kindly man with a moustache entering the room.

Operant conditioning

Operant conditioning is essentially different because it is the way voluntary behaviours (as opposed to reflexes) become associated with stimuli. It is describes the process by which behaviours are 'shaped' by whether they are reinforced (rewarded) or not. The basic idea is that we are more likely to repeat a behaviour if something good happens immediately after every time (or most times) we do it. B.F. Skinner conducted the pioneering experiments where he automated the whole process of training rats and pigeons to do a range of things, in his 'Skinner Box', by giving them food pellets as rewards immediately afterwards.

Skinner had no time for colleagues who wanted to label people 'normal' or 'abnormal', 'sane' or 'crazy'. He preferred to understand our differences in terms of our personal history of what had and had not been reinforced. In very simplistic terms, a shy person with great difficulty making friends would be understood as not having had many social skills reinforced (they would have a 'behavioural deficit'), while someone who does 'bad' or 'mad' things will have learned those behaviours by being rewarded for them somewhere along the line. When we say 'learned', we must realise that life presents us with many situations that resemble a Skinner Box. So if a person gains relief from voices in their head by shouting back at them, you can see how behaviour perceived by others as 'mad' might be learned. If we take the trouble to discover a person's history, we might understand their 'strange' behaviour. Other psychological models might help us understand why they hear voices in the first place.

All parents are using 'operant conditioning' every time they praise their children for being helpful or polite without realising there is a scientific name for it. Most people instinctively recognise the value of rewarding certain behaviours and ignoring the behaviours you don't want. It works. It's important to note that Skinner and others clearly demonstrated that the way to get rid of unwanted behaviour is a process of 'extinction' or lack of reinforcement. The application of aversive stimuli – popularly known as punishment – does not extinguish unwanted behaviour. It only suppresses it until the punishment stops. People who advocate the 'carrot and stick' have only got it half right. The carrot works but the stick doesn't.

Operant conditioning might apply to the causes of mental health problems. For example:

• Depression can be thought of as a general lack of reinforcement. For human beings a reinforcement is, by definition, something that makes us feel *good*. If nothing good happens to us for a long period of time, no matter what we try to do, we start doing less and less. The less we do, the fewer rewards we receive, and the more depressed we get. So we can get into a downward spiral of doing less and less and feeling worse and worse. This suggests that the cure for this is to force ourselves (perhaps with the help of a friend) to do something, anything, however trivial, that makes us feel good. Gradually, and with a lot of effort at first, we can start to remember what it is like to feel good (even for a couple of minutes) and we then have a little more energy to do a little more, which makes us feel a little better, and thus we can replace the downward spiral with an upwards one – but it takes more effort than staying depressed or drowning our sorrows in bottles of pills or alcohol.

• Gambling addiction is easily understood once we understand that certain 'schedules of reinforcement' are particularly hard to 'extinguish'. Skinner showed that after a behaviour has become established through repeated reinforcement it can be extinguished by removing the reward. After a few repetitions of pressing the bar the rat learns that the food pellet no longer arrives and stops pressing. However if the original learning had involved a schedule of reinforcement (the relationship between how many times the bar is pressed by the rat in order to get one pellet of food) where it's impossible to predict when the food will arrive (i.e., every so often with no pattern to it) then the bar-pressing behaviour becomes extremely difficult to extinguish. This is the type of reinforcement schedule programmed into slot and gaming machines and the responses (putting the money in and pulling the handle) are very difficult to stop – just one more press, the next one might be the one!

So learning theory places great emphasis on our environment, on the events and people that shape our behaviour. We are all reinforcing, ignoring or punishing one another all the time. It is how we get what we want from one another and negotiate the world. It could be that some of us have had things reinforced too often that make us uncomfortable or distressed or haven't had the things that help us feel joyful and fulfilled reinforced enough.

Social learning theory

Of the many ideas that come under this general heading, we have chosen two that we think might be particularly helpful when trying to understand the causes of our emotional difficulties: observational learning and self-reinforcement.

Observational learning is just a fancy term for copying other people. You don't need to be a psychologist to know that a lot of how we behave or feel is simply the result of imitating others – often automatically, without knowing we are doing it. It could originate from the fact that we humans, like many other animals, are social creatures and must learn to fit in with what goes on around us.

Any parent of a teenager understands just how powerful an influence peer pressure can be, as we feel our own influence beginning to fade away. However, peer pressure actually starts much earlier than that. As children we all copy mum and dad, or older brothers and sisters, then school friends and even teachers and so on. Observational learning is essentially copying what we have seen without actually being reinforced. We just do it because we have seen it. Other experiments have found the perhaps equally obvious fact that we are particularly likely to copy certain types of people, especially powerful people, those we like or respect, or those we want to be like. We are all familiar with the term 'role model'; it's just that young people refuse to choose the right ones!

So when trying to understand how you respond when life throws hard stuff at you, have a think about how mum and dad (or whoever your earliest 'role model' was) dealt with hard stuff. When you do this it becomes obvious why it is silly to assume that just because depression, or psychosis, or anxiety or whatever 'runs in families' the best way to understand that is to start looking at genes. Our patterns of how we respond when bad things happen to us (or when good things don't) often go back several generations. Where do you think your dad learned to be the way he was? Who had he copied?

Albert Bandura conducted a famous experiment in which children observed an adult behaving violently towards a large child-sized skittle-like doll which bounced back upright when hit or kicked. When the children were allowed back in the playroom, they imitated the adult's violent behaviour. This became known as 'vicarious learning', 'observational learning' or 'modelling', the interesting feature being that the young children were not actively rewarded to copy the adult's behaviour. They just seemed to do it naturally. This finding from Bandura leads to the social learning theory idea that rather than just being passive victims of reinforcements in our early childhoods, we continually set ourselves goals and can reinforce, or punish, *ourselves* for our progress, or lack thereof, towards those goals. While psychoanalysis and behaviourism may feel good as explanations because we are less responsible for the messes we get into, the social learning theory notion is a bit more challenging as we have to accept more responsibility. The idea is that we can, to a large extent, set our own compass and help ourselves move in our chosen direction by praising ourselves for any progress. This 'self-talk' idea overlaps with cognitive theory which we will cover next.

Cognitive theory

Psychologists were not too interested in thoughts when behaviourism was at its height in academic psychology. Measuring what goes on in the 'black box' or privacy of our own skulls was extremely difficult (if not heresy) and so didn't pass muster as real 'science'. Cognitive psychology (the study of thought processes) did thrive during and after World War II, but mainly by way of helping us understand the sort of mistakes people made when looking at radar screens or when having to make a decision after being on duty for 48 hours without a break. It wasn't until the 1960s that Aaron Beck pressed cognitive theory into practice as a model for psychological distress. Albert Ellis, originator of Rational Emotive Behaviour Therapy, was another pioneer of this approach, developing detailed theory and practice protocols.

When first encountering cognitive therapy some people

find the idea of changing people's thoughts at least disrespectful, possibly brutal, or in extreme cases, a version of mind control. However, like so many things pressed into practice to help someone who is desperate, in the hands of a good, sensitive practitioner, patients and clients experience it as informative, helpful, even liberating.

The basic model is wonderfully simple. Usually when a depressing thing happens we feel depressed. What has caused the feeling? Obviously the depressing event. Not necessarily, argue the cognitive theorists. Their evidence is that, faced with the same event, not all of us will be equally depressed, and some of us won't be the slightest bit bothered. What makes the difference? What we tell ourselves about the event, or about ourselves. This is the A-B-C model, where A is the event, C is the feeling that follows the event, and B – the all-important factor – is our thoughts.

The following example might help explain the process. After weeks of trying to get up the courage, you finally ask someone you have long had your eye on out on a date. To your astonishment they agree. You agree to meet outside a cinema. The big day arrives. You arrive on time and you wait, and wait and … you go home feeling down. Wouldn't everyone feel the same? The answer is no. It depends on many things – such as how many times this has happened before. But a major determinant is that little voice inside you trying to make sense of it all. You can tell yourself it's because you are ugly, because you are somehow just unlovable. You can tell yourself you'll never have a girlfriend or boyfriend. The list of ways to do yourself in is endless. Or you could assume there was a plausible reason the other person didn't show, because something has happened to interrupt their plans, travel and so on. Or you could even convince yourself that anyone not together enough to realise that you were the best catch around wasn't worth bothering with!

The thing is most of us have one or two 'negative self-statements' we use to bash ourselves over the heads with whenever something goes wrong. They are different for each of us but whichever ones we are burdened with, they are like a little close-looped audiotape lurking just below the surface of consciousness waiting to be triggered by something, anything, bad happening. We have our ready-made explanation.

John's main one used to be (and on a bad day still is) that he is stupid, dumb, unintelligent. It played itself in different keys – including 'if you weren't so thick you would have known that would happen' – but the melody was always the same. Cognitive therapy is designed to help us catch these thoughts. This is not easy because they happen automatically and often without awareness, which is why a cognitive therapist will ask you to keep a thought diary. If you can catch your own particular way of putting yourself down, the next step is to start the work of replacing it with something a little more helpful and realistic. Not 'I am Albert Einstein', but perhaps 'I am sometimes quite clever'.

But, as we have reminded ourselves before, this book is about causes not treatments. Readers wanting an honest evaluation of psychological treatments could look at David Pilgrim's book in this series *A Straight Talking Introduction to Psychological Treatments for Mental Health Problems.* Cognitive theory suggests that mental health problems are caused by our inaccurate and negative thoughts about ourselves, about the world, about the future and so on. That is an idea that most readers will be able to identify with. But without exploring where the ideas came from in the first place you can end up being even more hard on yourself with statements like 'Oh my god, not only am I depressed, obsessive, alcoholic, anxious – I am also one of those people who has negative self-statements!'

To understand the causes of mental health problems from a cognitive perspective you need to try and discover where the 'cognitions' came from. How, for instance, did someone like John – who was almost always top of his class – end up telling himself he was stupid. Well, like you, he learned his own special way of putting himself down early in life. Many people discover that the negative self-talk, the words going round in circles in their heads waiting to be released by some unfortunate incident, are the words of a teacher or parent or someone else important to them in some way who, perhaps in a moment of anger, (or several moments of anger) said something about you that wasn't very nice. And it got stuck there.

Cognitive therapy practitioners would want us to explain that cognitive therapy is much more complicated than how we have described it above, but with limited space we cannot do justice to *any* of the theories we are summarising. Nevertheless we will mention just one or two of the complexities.

Firstly, it isn't just *what* we think that matters. *How* we think can be important too. We tend to develop *patterns* of thinking and some of these can cause us problems. Some examples include:

Selective abstraction Focusing only on the negative aspects of a situation. For example, the one thing you forgot to do today, rather than all the things you did remember to do.

Overgeneralisation Drawing big conclusions on the basis of a single, small, event. Assuming that because you were late for work today you are an incompetent or unvalued worker.

Magnification and minimisation Exaggerating bad things about ourselves while downplaying the positives.

All-or-nothing thinking Seeing events or people (including ourselves) as either all bad or all good. For example, putting people into our 'good box' or 'bad box' within a few seconds of meeting them (or before we have even met them at all).

Personalisation Assuming that we are always responsible for other people's feelings. For instance, believing that just because your partner is upset you must have done something wrong. (Maybe you did of course, but try finding out.)

So, when a bad thing happens, we have some choices about what we tell ourselves. There are at least three dimensions to the 'attributions' we make about a bad event. These are internal–external, global–specific, and permanent–temporary. If John's students want to feel really depressed the next time they get a bad grade they should tell themselves: (1) that the grade was caused by something about themselves (internal) – being thick will do; (2) that this is a global phenomenon – they are thick at everything not just psychology; and (3) that this is permanent – they always have been and always will be thick. Alternatively they could brighten up their day a bit by going external (Dr Read set an unfair exam); specific (other lecturers don't do that); and temporary (even though this one was unfair, Dr Read's exams are usually fair so this won't happen again).

There are two potential problems in looking at things this way. Firstly, there is a risk of blaming yourself for blaming yourself if you don't figure out where the blaming started. Secondly, sometimes life really *is* depressing. Sometimes it *isn't* what we tell ourselves about an event, it really is the event itself (or a series of events) that is the cause of our problems. So we have to be careful that we don't go to the other extreme of living with rose-tinted glasses on, denying that there is some pretty awful stuff going on sometimes, to ourselves and to those around us. In fact there are a few studies that show that when we are depressed we actually see some aspects of the world (including how others judge us) more accurately than people who are not depressed![8,9] Having said that, many have found this cognitive approach to be really good when it comes to helping figure out why we don't like ourselves as much as we should.

Humanistic theory

Abraham Maslow (1908–1970) is often cited as the founder of humanistic psychology. In common with the other approaches, it's difficult to summarise in a page or two, but in the case of humanistic psychology this is because there are so many different approaches underneath the umbrella term. The ideas were developed in the mid-20th century based on the contemporary philosophies of existentialism[10] and phenomenology,[11] and focusing on the prime human qualities of hope, love, creativity and the central importance of lived experience.

The revolutionary idea that people could help themselves – Person-Centred Therapy

Maslow's ideas did not translate into a therapeutic approach, but American psychologist Carl Rogers (1902–1982) developed a theory of distress and a therapeutic method which influenced psychology worldwide. Some of Rogers' ideas are, like Freud's, so influential that they have been incorporated into psychological therapies so successfully that they are practically taken as read and have become a sort of therapeutic commonsense.

The name of Rogers' approach changed over the years, and the way this happened says something about both the man and the approach. In the late 1930s and throughout the 1940s, Rogers developed his approach from his experiences working with patients, initially with 'problem children'. Two key principles in his early work were (i) to rely on the individual's own tendency towards growth (getting better) and (ii) to not interfere too much in this or 'play the expert'. He started to call this method 'non-directive therapy' to emphasise the importance of acknowledging the idea that if supported appropriately, people could find solutions to their own problems.

By 1951, Rogers was calling the approach 'client-centred therapy' to give more emphasis to the notion that the 'client' (rather than the medical term 'patient') was the expert in their own lives and that the therapist was in their service. Soon he changed the name one final time to 'person-centred therapy' to address even more of the power imbalance between the person wanting help and the person offering help as a companion. He was set against expertism and was convinced that people really could grow positively through distress if provided with the right conditions.[12]

The causes of distress – Conditional love and being 'incongruent'

Rogers' theory is easy to oversimplify and make it sound ridiculous. It has a very 'commonsense' feel to it and at the same time has several components which set it against almost all other theories and many accepted practices in mental health services. In a nutshell, he stated that human infants (and adults for that matter) need unconditional acceptance in order to grow (and maintain) a healthy self-structure. Every time they are offered *conditional* love (on the basis that they behave in a certain way) they build up a set of ideas about themselves based not on their own experiences, but on the values and judgements of others. Here Rogers is talking about a very wide range of things from, e.g., sexuality (only loved and accepted if you are straight) through to expression of thoughts and feelings (only loved if you keep quiet about abuse). Also note that this withholding of love can be unspoken and very subtle, or quite brutal.

This results in an 'imported' self-structure which starts to operate separately from the person's natural ability to experience the world for themselves, and when these two elements are in conflict he called this 'incongruence'. If a person has a lot of imported material (rather than that based on self-evaluated experience) they experience more and more unpleasant conflict between these two parts of themselves as they go about their everyday life experiencing the world. It is easy to see how these internalised judgemental (or self-sustaining) elements can become experienced as 'voices'.

Some experiences will be congruent in that they 'fit' the person's view of themselves (I am gay and being attracted to men feels good) but many will not fit and are experienced as a threat to the whole of the self-structure (I have these feelings which are wrong – I am bad and unlovable). Since incongruent experiences suggest that either the experience or the self-structure is 'wrong', something has to give. Either the person denies or distorts the experience (to make it fit), or they suffer from anxiety (anything from a relentless niggling discomfort to a panic attack), which in turn is an experience which may not fit with their image of themselves (I'm a positive person, not someone who feels afraid all the time).

The more your personality is determined by the judgemental influence of others the more discrepancy between your experiences and your self-image there will be. The more discrepancy there is, the more threatened your self-structure will be. We naturally fortify our wobbly self-structure by making it more solid and rigid (ironically, trying to support the elements within it that are causing the problem in the first place). A healthy self-structure needs to be flexible, since life unfolds in unexpected ways and we must respond creatively, not with the same old rigid patterns.

If threatened enough (e.g., trying to deny or distort past abuse, or defend against trauma, loss, or unremitting stress) the brittle self-structure will eventually break and loss of identity and/or chaotic thinking and feeling will result.

Since the fault lines in the self-structure were caused initially by judgemental, conditional love, 'treatment' is intended to offer a therapeutic relationship 'involving primarily complete absence of any threat to the self-structure'.[13] If this can be sustained, this will lead to the person 'self-righting' and the fault lines sealed with new, trustworthy self-accredited experiences. If a superficial quick fix is applied, the fault lines remain, ready to be activated by new challenging life experiences.

What is so different about this approach is that person-centred theory says that there is a single type of cause for all distress. This single cause, though, finds an unlimited number of ways of expressing itself because each person and their lived experience is different. This makes any one person's trajectory of distress completely unpredictable unless their effort is turned 100% to finding the meaning of the experiences with the best expert available – the person themself. Such a theory is completely antagonistic to any kind of system of categories or diagnosis, including the medical model. It also means that person-centred literature is not crowded with books and articles on how to differentially treat this problem or that diagnosis. For professionals who think that complicated diagnostic categories and expert-driven treatment protocols are a sign of sophistication, this leaves the person-centred approach looking lightweight and naïve.

Before Rogers, professional therapy relationships were

cast in the mould of the powerful expert doctor and helpless patient lacking insight. Rogers' work made it possible for lay people (non-medically qualified) and other professionals to work much more as companions in a person-to-person way – something which many of us now see as essential (but, sadly, still cannot be taken for granted). Rogers was not only a pioneer of the importance of the relationship in therapy, he was the first to record a complete therapy relationship onto wax discs, publish a word-for-word transcript and initiate research into the effectiveness of psychotherapy, including looking at individual interventions.[14,15]

Conclusion

We hope this brief trip through some of the theories might help you to figure out some new ways to think about your problems, or those of a loved one. Or maybe one or two of them just confirm what you already thought. We suggest you don't try too hard to pick the best theory. There is a lot of overlap between them. For example – are the defence mechanisms that Freud talks about really so different from the 'faulty thinking' described by the cognitive theorists? They are both examples of how we distort or misperceive ourselves and the world around us. Perhaps all the theories have something to offer at different times in your life. If there is a common message it is perhaps that we aren't born with the problems we have as adults, they aren't somehow inherently and inevitably built into our brains; they come from our interactions with other people, especially, but not exclusively, early on in life.

We now move on to look at how the causes identified in Chapter 6 and the theories discussed here apply to the most common problem of all, experienced by most of us at some time in our lives – depression.

Chapter 8
An example of putting things together: Formulating depression

What is formulation?

Formulation is the process that an increasing number of mental health professionals use to put together and make sense of the information they gather during formal assessment and other sources in order to create a systematic, positive framework of action to help the client. A crucial element of formulation is positively acting upon the fact that for many clients, their own understanding of the difficulties that they or their relatives experience can be the key to making positive changes in their lives.

For many professionals, formulation is replacing diagnosis as the main framework for making sense of their clients' experiences. One of the aims is to empower people by identifying, in partnership with them, areas for change and development. This is in contrast to simple diagnosis and prescription of treatment which often leaves people feeling dependent on professionals to solve their difficulties.

Developing understanding by using formulation as a method

In order to show how the causes, listed in Chapter 6, and the psychological theories, described in Chapter 7, can work together to create a 'mental health problem', an example may be helpful. We thought it would be a good idea to continue with our example of depression. It is the most common diagnosis in the diagnostic manual. One in six people in the UK will suffer from an experience which would be classified as depression at some point in their life. According to the 2003 WHO fact sheet on mental health in Europe, 33.4 million people in the region suffer from depression in any given year, and more than 30 million people in the world have now been prescribed the antidepressant Prozac. In addition many people whose primary problem is something else (anxiety, eating disorders, drug and alcohol problems, psychosis etc.) are also thought to be 'depressed'.

Diagnosis is not a formulation
Many psychiatrists argue that there is a difference between ordinary depression or sadness and what they call 'major depression' which they consider to be a 'mental illness'. *The Diagnostic and Statistical Manual* (DSM – see Chapter 4) has a way of separating those who just feel depressed and those who have this thing called 'Major Depressive Disorder' (MDD). It does so by what some have called the 'smorgasbord approach to diagnosis'. This involves listing some behaviours and feelings and then saying you need a certain number of them to be categorised as having the thing in question. To be labelled as having MDD you need any five of the following nine 'symptoms':

- depressed mood
- loss of interest in things that normally give you pleasure
- weight loss or gain
- sleeping difficulties
- agitation or slowing down of movement responses
- fatigue or loss of energy

- feelings of worthlessness or guilt
- concentration or decision-making difficulties
- suicidal thoughts

For this particular diagnosis you need to have had these five (or more) symptoms for most of the time almost every day, for a two-week period.

A diagnosis from an appropriately qualified mental health professional can be useful for managers of mental health services who have to decide how to allocate limited resources. In some countries it is *essential* if the person is to access services or funding for services. Those with a diagnosis like MDD are, therefore, likely to get help; those who do not meet the criteria (with, say, only four out of nine 'symptoms') are unlikely to get help. But this process is useless when it comes to deciding whether a person is 'actually depressed' or not. The real world of human emotions does not fit into nice little boxes and, as we hope we have shown in previous chapters, they are incredibly difficult to define, in terms of generalised experience. Depression (and anxiety and most other problems) is not a category of experience that anyone can say with confidence that some of us have and some of us do not. At best it is a dimension or continuum of experience along which we all vary from month to month, day to day and sometimes even hour to hour. Naturally we would expect some folk to have a broader range of movement up and down this dimension. And others spend too much time down in the more depressed end of the dimension. But to claim that some of us *have* some*thing* called 'depression' and some of us don't is an argument that's difficult to sustain.

If we believe we *have* something called 'depression' or 'MDD' then it's all too easy to start also believing that this thing, this disorder or mental illness, is actually somehow *causing* us to feel depressed. People who think like this are likely to answer the question 'Why are you feeling depressed?' with 'Because I have MDD'. Regardless of the lack of logic, we are invited to believe that the symptoms in the list used to decide who has this thing called MDD are supposedly caused by the label given to people who have five or more. For example 'Different people are affected in different ways by major depression. Some people have trouble sleeping, they lose weight, and they generally feel agitated and irritable.' This is a circular argument that actually explains nothing about the causes of the experiences which we might label as feeling depressed. It does create a situation where everyone concerned (from the person in question through to the mental health professionals working with them) need not bother to try to figure out what has really caused them to feel so down and what changes might be needed (in thinking, feeling, behaviour or living conditions) in order to feel better. Some people are happy with this sort of approach to understanding the causes of 'depression', since the reassurance (we repeat, regardless of the lack of logic) is comforting.

Sources of information

Biological theories

In recent years depression, like everything else, has received much attention from genetic researchers. There is evidence that depression runs in families.[1] There is also evidence that when people are depressed the neurotransmitters (especially serotonin and norepinephrine) are either at a low level or are out of balance with each other,[2] and metabolism is slower in certain parts of the brain.[3]

We have already argued, however, that just because problems, including depression, run in families does not mean there is a genetic component. It can be depressing growing up with depressed parents – either because mum and dad are too preoccupied or sad to give us what we need as kids and/or because we learn to copy their way of dealing with problems. We have also, however, argued that everything is an interaction between our genes and our environment. We just don't believe there is any good evidence that there is a specific genetic predisposition to specific mental health problems. Probably the most important thing we inherit is a greater or lesser sensitivity to stress in general. But even so it is hard to say, at birth for instance, what is genetic and what is the result of mum being stressed during pregnancy. We have also argued, too, that there isn't a whole lot we can do about our genetic makeup and that it is more useful, therefore, to focus on the depressing things (and our reactions to them) that have caused our depression and figure out which ones we can do something about.

We have also already argued that just because our brains function differently when we are depressed that does not mean there is something wrong with our brains that has somehow caused 'the depression'. Our brains are simply responding to depressing events.

External causes

In Chapter 6 we looked at some of the research studies proving that the public is right (Chapter 5) to assume that depression (like other mental health problems) is primarily caused by depressing things happening in our lives. For example, you may remember the 2007 study covering 14 USA states which found that admission to hospital for depression was significantly predicted by poverty and unemployment.[4] Other environmental or external events that can help cause depression include: child abuse (emotional, physical and sexual), child neglect, bullying in schools, violence including rape, being an immigrant or member of an ethic minority (especially if poor and/or you experience discrimination) and loss.

Loss, of course, is a strong candidate as a cause of depression. We have seen (in Chapter 6) that loss comes in many shapes and sizes and is an inevitable part of being human. We have discussed why some people who experience, for instance, the loss of a cherished partner or a job they valued, seem to cope with the sadness and others seem to get stuck in a very deep feeling of hopelessness about the future. Some of the things that make the difference are other external factors including previous losses, level of support from friends and family, our general quality of life beyond who or what we have just lost. We have also seen, however, that internal factors, including what we tell ourselves about the loss, are also hugely important.

Internal causes

Believing (for whatever reason) that your feelings are caused by an imagined irreversible chemical imbalance in your brain, or faulty genes, or a 'mental illness' called 'Major Depressive Disorder', whilst possibly reassuring, is not particularly motivating. Empowering individual people in their struggle with distress and disturbing experiences is a tricky thing – balancing reassurance and hope with challenging 'home truths'. We have explained that we understand why so many people find diagnosis reassuring or even a lifeline in desperate times, but we are convinced that simply diagnosing experiences using arbitrary labels is unhelpful in the long run. Some beliefs are born out of our efforts to cope with our experiences – some of these will be helpful and some will not be. In truth it's very difficult for anyone on the 'outside' of the experiences to know what will be helpful to any particular client. The skill is to work in a consultative partnership with the client to find out what helps, what hinders, what is harmful and what is positive. In the summary of the cognitive theory in Chapter 7 we looked at a range of other unhelpful things we tell ourselves that can cause or exacerbate feeling depressed.

Amongst many mental health professions, cognitive theory has become a very popular way to understand and treat depression (see Chapter 7). Blaming ourselves when depressing things happen is all too easy to do – especially when we are little. At certain stages in their emotional and cognitive development, children tend to think everything is to do with themselves. So as a child, when anything bad (or good for that matter) happens we think we must be responsible. If Mummy and Daddy split up, as a five year old we could easily assume that it was something we did, or didn't do, that caused it, unless they went out of their way to explain otherwise and demonstrate it in their behaviour. Grownups can also sometimes have a tendency to feel overly responsible for things.

Although cognitive theory can be helpful in understanding and overcoming depression, other theories can help our understanding as well. In terms of psychodynamic and humanistic theories, we might ask whether our parents were so focused on teaching us right from wrong that they forgot to make sure we felt loved for ourselves. Did they give us the impression that they only loved us if we achieved well at school, or fulfilled their aspirations for us? Attachment theory would have us consider if events in early life meant that we couldn't establish a safe, trusting relationship in our first few years.

Did we learn early on in life, from our main role models, to withdraw from others and close down emotionally whenever something depressing happens as might be suggested by social learning theory? Or did we simply learn to stop doing the things which make us feel good when we first start feeling a bit down – producing a downward spiral?

Positives as well as negatives
There is a tendency amongst mental health professionals to focus on the negative. First we list all the 'pathological' behaviours or thoughts that someone has and then, having applied the appropriate label, we go in search of bad things to explain the bad behaviours – whether they be dysfunctional brains, faulty genes, unhappy childhoods or what have you. Life is not really like that. Life is, of course, a combination of good and bad. So when trying to understand another human being (or ourselves) we need to factor in the positives. From a practical point of view, in terms of what helps when we are depressed, it can be very important to focus on our existing strengths, so they can be valued and nurtured, as well as on the things (external and internal) that we might want to change. A famous psychologist, George Albee, came up with a rather simple equation for thinking about the chances of developing depression or other mental health problems. [5]

$$\text{Chances of mental health problem} = \frac{\text{Organic factors} + \text{Stress} + \text{Exploitation}}{\text{Coping skills} + \text{Self-esteem} + \text{Support groups}}$$

More recent authors, writing about how to prevent psychosis, added:

To reduce the incidence of madness, we must increase the size of the denominator [below the line] and decrease the size of the numerator [above the line]. This requires reducing our exposure to stressful or traumatic events and increasing our capacity to participate fully in the world by creating a more just society. At the same time, it involves increasing our ability to cope with trauma and inequity, by learning better coping skills, enhancing our self-esteem and developing better formal and informal social support systems.[6]

Putting it all together – the formulation

In training programmes across a range of disciplines around the world, students are taught to 'formulate' – to attempt to put all the information about a person's mental health problem together. So far in this chapter we have tried to put some flesh on the bones of the idea that the type of formulation you come up with depends on what sort of information you have got to work with and what sort of model you have in mind. As we suggested at the start of the chapter, if you are working from a 'medical model' and only know what 'symptoms' a person has, you come up with nothing more than a 'diagnostic formulation' which is a fancy term for a label. If, however, you have taken a thorough psychosocial history (covering the sorts of things discussed in Chapter 6), and you have some understanding of psychological theories (Chapter 7), you come up with something much more interesting and much more useful.

A psychological formulation tries to explain a problem like depression in terms of the person's life history. It tries, however, to go beyond just listing all the depressing things that have happened. The goal is to answer the question: *How* did those things lead to someone feeling hopeless about the future, etc? It is also, therefore, addressing the question of why, after the death of their husband, did *this* person, the client or patient in front of us, end up severely depressed when others who suffer a similar loss do not?

There are many ways to approach a formulation. One way is to break things down into Predisposing factors, Precipitating factors, Perpetuating factors and Preventative factors (the 'four Ps'). Predisposing factors tend to be things that happened earlier in life that increase the chances of getting very depressed when, later in life, a depressing thing happens (the precipitating factor). Predisposing factors can be external events – such as child abuse or early loss of a parent, but they include internal processes – such as learning early on in life to blame yourself for everything that goes wrong, to dislike yourself, to be scared of close relationships etc. A precipitating factor is anything that pushes you over the edge, sometimes by triggering one or more of your predisposing factors. So someone with a lot of early losses – or one huge early loss – can sometimes become very depressed when faced with another loss later in life. Perpetuating factors are, as the term implies, anything that tends to maintain the problem, such as chronic stressors, poverty, unsupportive family etc., or internal factors like telling yourself you are unlovable etc.). Preventative factors are the strengths that a person has despite all their problems, internal (skills and so on) and external (support from friends and family, a good job etc.).

Formulations are usually done at the level of the individual person, although it can be invaluable (although more complicated) to formulate a group, for instance, a family.

If you, or a loved one, are sometimes (or often) depressed, it might be helpful to try to list the predisposing, precipitating, perpetuating and preventive factors involved.

Some examples of the four Ps in relation to depression

Predisposing (in past)	Precipitating (recent)	Perpetuating (current/ ongoing)	Preventative (current/ ongoing)
External	*External*	*External*	*External*
childhood neglect	loss (person, job etc.)	no friends	supportive family
childhood abuse	failure	critical family/ friends	supportive friends
bullying	physical	work stress violence	satisfying job
depressed parent(s)	emotional abuse	unemploy- ment	children
deaths in family	financial problems	poverty	
other losses	other depress- ing events	parenting stress	
poverty			
discrimination			
Internal	*Internal*	*Internal*	*Internal*
blaming self for any of the above	realisation dreams or goals not being attained	hopeless about future	hope for the future
learning to distrust other people	humiliating failure at work	dislike of self	a plan
feeling loved only if we live up to others' expectations	failure of relationship	fear of other people	liking self

Then, using one or more of the models (pick the ones that make most sense to you – or make up your own 'model'), try to fit it all together. The diagram below illustrates one possibility. There is no totally complete or correct formulation, so don't worry about getting it 'right'. It's a way of having a constructive dialogue with yourself about your experiences – some of the connections you make in undertaking this exercise may jump out at you as making sense.

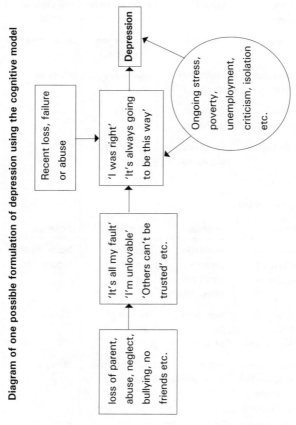

Diagram of one possible formulation of depression using the cognitive model

loss of parent, abuse, neglect, bullying, no friends etc.

'It's all my fault' 'I'm unlovable' 'Others can't be trusted' etc.

Recent loss, failure or abuse

'I was right' 'It's always going to be this way'

Ongoing stress, poverty, unemployment, criticism, isolation etc.

Depression

Of course many readers will have already been doing this for years. We all have our formulations of our problems (and other people's). We just don't call them formulations. Any case study submitted in training by a student that has a thorough and sensible formulation, but does not include the client's formulation, should be returned to them as incomplete. Mental health professionals often forget that clients (or 'patients' if you must) already have their own theories about what is causing, and maintaining, the problem. Sometimes, however, the client's formulation has been part of the problem – a perpetuating factor in its own right. If a client's formulation of why they feel depressed so much of the time is that they are somehow a bad person who deserves to feel so wretched, or that they have a mental illness called 'depressive disorder' about which nothing much can be done – then we think that needs some further thought. Some formulations are more helpful than others.

So while it simply can't be the case in mental health services that the 'customer is *always* right', it is absolutely essential that all practitioners (from support workers to consultant psychiatrists) *listen respectfully*. Being respectful includes sharing one's formulation with the client and then talking about any differences. There always are differences. Two heads are invariably better than one when trying to understand something as complicated as a human being – especially when one of the heads is the subject of the formulation. So, in trying to understand the causes of a person's 'depression' we think good practice requires the professional to ask the patient or client to construct their own 'formulation'. If you are reading this book and wondering about whether your own experiences would add up to a diagnosis of 'depression', why not try your own formulation? Then check it out with a couple of people who know you well – what do they think? Make sure you choose these people well. They need to be people whose judgement you trust but also who are able to be honest with you. Don't take their views as 'the truth' – just one more perspective to be taken into consideration.

A word of caution

If you are reading this book in order to gain a better understanding of your own experiences or of someone close to you, it's worthwhile proceeding with caution. A quick look at the table on p. 135 should be enough to make us realise that we all have a range of precipitating factors and for some of us, that list will include thinking about our problems. How sensitive we are to thoughts as precipitating factors will depend on us as individuals. We all react in different ways. For some it will be a positive, empowering discovery, for others it might be a trigger for a mildly disturbing, but handleable experience and for a few it might be akin to reliving a trauma or abuse.

If you can guess beforehand that trying your own formulation will trigger disturbance or distress or re-traumatise you, either don't do it or attempt it only with support from a trusted friend or professional.

Chapter 9
Keep thinking (and feeling) about the causes of mental health problems

We have seen that there are lots of possible reasons why some of us sometimes feel extremely overwhelmed, frightened, distressed, depressed or confused. There are also lots of different theories about *how* this long list of events can operate on us, and in us, to bring about these problems. Perhaps that is the most important lesson from all this: that there is no one correct answer to the question of what causes mental health problems. And the lesson resulting from *that* is that we should be wary of anyone, expert or friend, who tells us they know what is the cause of our problem, especially if they tell us that one thing alone (biological, social *or* psychological) is the cause.

Genes, brain chemicals, child abuse, even the most painful early loss, are not by themselves likely to be the whole answer. It is usually a combination of things, past and present, external and internal. It is complicated, but not so complicated that it isn't worth trying to figure out the major factors and how they may be interacting. You stand a good chance of finding out some of the causes, and in almost all cases will learn something potentially useful. However, this involves not only a bit of thinking but, often, some feeling too. Digging around in the past is not always pleasant. Perhaps that is why diagnoses and simplistic biological theories are so attractive. They are not only simple, they are also relatively pain free.

So, when *thinking* about the causes of mental health problems, sometimes patients and clients have to be prepared to do some *feeling* too. Sometimes the thoughts and feelings they discover will turn out to be not 'mental health problems' at all, just understandable emotional reactions to things that have happened. And sometimes they must avoid falling into the trap of believing that it was *all* horrible. It might also be the case that they need to do a little more work on *accepting* certain feelings as normal and a little less work on *changing* – which may come from labelling something a 'problem'. So, paradoxically, and in contrast to our 'word of caution' section on p. 138, thinking about the causes of 'mental health problems' can sometimes get rid of the 'problem' all by itself.

One of the dilemmas in all this was illustrated by the research (Chapter 7) showing that when we are depressed we sometimes see the world more accurately than when we are happy. So to some extent you have to decide, for yourself, whether it is better to be happy or wise.

Of course people sometimes need to do something more than just accept that *most* people would have reacted the way they did under the same circumstances. In that case having a good understanding of what factors, in the world around them and in their own minds, have contributed, and which ones may still be contributing, is a great place to start when deciding what course of action to take. Professionals need to be aware of these possibilities too – if the cause is an environmental factor, it will probably be worthwhile trying to change the environment.

Thinking about the causes of mental health problems may not only help us accept or change ourselves; we could end up doing our own small part, one way or another, to change that small bit of the world we have some influence over. We imagine many readers will be already doing that anyway.

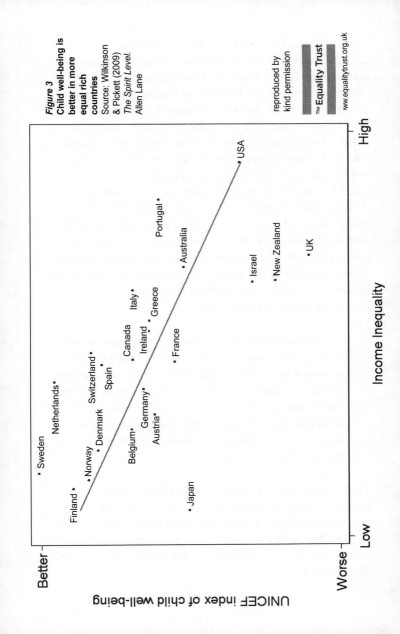

Figure 3
Child well-being is better in more equal rich countries
Source: Wilkinson & Pickett (2009) *The Spirit Level.* Allen Lane

UNICEF index of child well-being

Better

Worse

Income Inequality

Low

High

Sweden

Netherlands

Finland

Norway

Denmark

Switzerland

Spain

Belgium

Germany

Austria

Canada

Italy

Ireland

Greece

France

Japan

Australia

Portugal

Israel

New Zealand

UK

USA

Even though it would have been frustrating for us to say this at the outset, we hope we have provided more questions than answers in this book. Acknowledging how little we collectively know is the first step in finding out something worth saying about the causes of mental health problems.

And so we end with one more question regarding the causes of psychological distress. What does it mean when the World Health Organization says that one in four of us will have a mental disorder at some point in our lives?[1] In Great Britain, for example, in 2004 one in ten already had a clinically diagnosable mental disorder by age 16![2] The figures seem to be steadily increasing all over the world. Is it time we started to think about what role the societies we live in play in this huge and apparently increasing amount of human unhappiness and distress, and what we can do to prevent the causes of mental health problems?

George Albee put it this way:

> Psychologists must join with persons who reject racism, sexism, colonialism, and exploitation and must find ways to redistribute social power and to increase social justice. Primary prevention research inevitably will make clear the relationship between social pathology and psychopathology and then will work to change social and political structures in the interests of social justice. It is as simple and as difficult as that![3]

The focus on *relative* poverty should not be forgotten when planning primary prevention programmes. Figure 3 on p. 141 shows the relationship between inequality and the 'Index of child wellbeing in rich countries', a measure combining 40 indicators compiled by UNICEF. The authors of *The Spirit Level* conclude:

The solution to problems caused by inequality is not mass psychotherapy aimed at making everyone less vulnerable. The best way of responding to the harm done by high levels of inequality would be to reduce the inequality itself. Rather than requiring anti-anxiety drugs in the water supply or mass psychotherapy, what is most exciting about the picture we present is that it shows that reducing inequality would increase the wellbeing and quality of life for all of us.[4]

Endnotes

Chapter 1

1. See, for example, Remafedi, G, French, S, Story, M, Resnick, MD & Blum, R (1998) The relationship between suicide risk and sexual orientation: Results of a population-based study. *American Journal of Public Health* 88, 57–60.

2. And Ryan, C, Huebner, D, Diaz, RM & Sanchez, J (2009) Family rejection as a predictor of negative health outcomes in white and Latino lesbian, gay, and bisexual young adults. *Pediatrics, 123*(1), 346–52.

3. Kutchins, H & Kirk, SA (1999) Making Us Crazy: DSM – The psychiatric Bible and the creation of mental disorders. London: Constable.

4. *The Diagnostic and Statistical Manual of Mental Disorders* published by the American Psychiatric Association. Now in its fourth revised edition. DSM-III-R refers to the third revised edition published in 1987.

5. http://madpride.org.uk/index.php

6. Pilgrim, D (2009) *A Straight Talking Introduction to Psychological Treatments for Mental Health Problems*. Ross-on-Wye: PCCS Books.

7. *The Diagnostic and Statistical Manual of Mental Disorders*, fourth revised edition published by the American Psychiatric Association in 2000. The 'TR' stands for 'text revision'.

Chapter 2

1. Bynum, WF, Porter, R & Shepherd, M (eds) (1985) *The Anatomy of Madness*. London: Tavistock.

2. Porter, R (2002) *Madness: A brief history*. Oxford: Oxford University Press.

3. Shorter, A (1997) *History of Psychiatry: From the era of the asylum to the age of Prozac*. New York: John Wiley and Sons.

4. Page 19 in Alexander, F & Selesnick, S (1996) *The History of Psychiatric Thought and Practice from Prehistoric Times to the Present*. New York: Harper and Row.

5. Miller, N (1975) Israel and the Jews. In J Howells (ed) *World History of Psychiatry* (pp 528–46). New York: Brunner/Mazel.

6. Rosen, G (1964) *Madness in Society*. Chicago: University of Chicago Press.

7. Deuteronomy 28: 28.

8. Deuteronomy 28: 34.

9. Leviticus 20: 27.

10. Deuteronomy 22: 22.

11. Read, J & Masson, J (2004) Genetics, eugenics and mass murder. In J Read, LR Mosher & R Bentall (eds) *Models of Madness* (pp 35–42). London: Routledge.

12. Page 529 in Miller, 1975. See n. 5.

13. Page 69 in Rosen, 1964. See n. 6.

14. Page 28 in Alexander & Selesnick, 1996. See n. 4.

15. Page xvii in Hippocrates (1931) *Sacred Heart* (trans. W Jones). London: Heinemann.

16. Ducey, C & Simon, B (1975) Ancient Greece and Rome. In J Howells (ed) *World History of Psychiatry* (pp 1–38). New York: Brunner/Mazel.

17. Page 19 in Ducey & Simon, 1975. See n. 16.

18. Page 21 in Ducey & Simon, 1975. See n. 16.

19. Page 916-c in Plato (1904) *Timaeus* (trans. R Bury). Cambridge, MA: Harvard University Press.

20. Page 43 in Kraemer, M & Sprenger, M (1486/1941) *Malleus Maleficarum* (trans. J Summer). London: Pushkin.

21. Michelet J (1939) *Satanism and Witchcraft*. Toronto: Citadel.

22. Page 47 in Kraemer & Sprenger, 1486/1941. See n. 20.

23. Page 108, 109 in Burton, R (1621/1961) *The Anatomy of Melancholy,* vol. 2. (F Dell & P Jourdan-Smith, eds). London: Dent.

24. Page 104 in Alexander & Selesnick, 1996. See n. 4.

25. Page 112 in Alexander & Selesnick, 1996. See n. 4.

26. Page 39 in Foucault, M (1965) *Madness and Civilisation*. New York: Random House.

27. Michel Foucault, French philosopher, sociologist and historian has written extensively on the history of madness. The phrase 'The Great Confinement' is taken from his book *Madness and Civilisation* (see n.26), the first *full* English translation is titled *The History of Madness,* published by Routledge in 2006.

28. Scull, A (1981) Moral treatment reconsidered. In A Scull (ed) *Madhouses, Mad-Doctors and Madmen* (pp 105–88). Philadelphia: University of Philadelphia.

29. Page 258 in Foucault, 1965. See n. 26.

30. Page 121 in Tuke S (1813) *Description of the Retreat.* York: Society of Friends.

31. Reil, J (1803) *Rhapsodien uber die Anwendung der Psychischen Curmethode auf Geisteszerruttungen*. Halle: Curt.

Chapter 3

1. See Watson, JB & Rayner, R, (1920) *Journal of Experimental Psychology*, 3(1), 1–14. This can be downloaded free from http://psychclassics.yorku.ca/Watson/emotion.htm on the excellent 'Classics in the History of Psychology' website. See also the 'All About Psychology' website: http://www.all-about-psychology.com

2. The work of BF Skinner can be found on the 'All About Psychology' website http://www.all-about-psychology.com and also 'Classics in the History of Pychology' website including this fascinating journal article about the development of superstition in pigeons (it's quite scientific) http://psychclassics.yorku.ca/Skinner/Pigeon

3. Retrieved 01/08/2010 from http://www.loc.gov/loc/brain/proclaim.html.

4. The Human Genome Project website: http://www.ornl.gov/sci/techresources/Human_Genome/home.shtml

5. Read, J, Fink, P, Rudegeair, T, Felitti, V & Whitfield, C (2008) Child maltreatment and psychosis: A return to a genuinely integrated bio-psycho-social model. *Clinical Schizophrenia and Related Psychoses, 7,* 235–54.

6. Read, J, Perry, B, Moskowitz, A & Connolly, J (2001) The contribution of early traumatic events to schizophrenia in some patients: A Traumagenic Neurodevelopmental model. *Psychiatry: Interpersonal and Biological Processes, 64,* 319–45.

7. Sanders, A, Duan, J, Levinson, D, Shi, J, He, D, Hou C et al. (2008) No significant association of 14 candidate genes with schizophrenia in a large European ancestry sample: Implications for psychiatric genetics. *Am J Psychiatry, 165*(4), 497–506.

8. Hamilton, S (2008) Schizophrenia candidate genes: Are we really coming up blank? *Am J Psychiatry, 165*(4), 420–3.

9. Rose, S (2005) *The 21st Century Brain: Explaining, mending and manipulating the mind.* London: Jonathan Cape.

10. Pages 144–5 in Bentall, RP (2009) *Doctoring the Mind: Why psychiatric treatments fail.* London: Penguin.

11. Champagne, F & Curley, J (2009) Epigenetic mechanisms mediating the long-term effects of maternal care on development. *Neuroscience and Biobehavioral Reviews, 33*, 593–600.

12. Read, J, Bentall, RP & Fosse, R (2009) Time to abandon the bio-bio-bio model of psychosis: Exploring the epigenetic and psychological mechanisms by which adverse life events lead to psychotic symptoms. *Epidemiologia e Psichiatria Sociale, 18*, 299–310.

13. Read, J & Masson, J (2004) Genetics, eugenics and mass murder. In J Read, LR Mosher & R Bentall (eds) *Models of Madness* (pp 35–42). London: Routledge.

14. Davies, E & Burdett, J (2004). Preventing 'schizophrenia': Creating the conditions for saner societies. In J Read, L Mosher L & R Bentall (eds) *Models of Madness* (pp 271–82). London: Routledge.

15. Mansell, P & Read, J (2009) The pharmaceutical industry and the Internet: Are drug company funded depression websites biased? *Journal of Mental Health, 10,* 9–23.

16. Read, J (2008) Schizophrenia, drug companies and the Internet. *Social Science & Medicine, 66,* 99–109.

17. De Wattignar, S & Read, J (2009) Posttraumatic stress disorder, drug companies and the Internet. *Journal of Trauma and Dissociation, 18,* 1–10.

18. Rampello, L, Nicoletti, F & Nicoletti, F (2000) Dopamine and depression: Therapeutic implications. *CNS Drugs, 13,* 35–45.

19. Janowsky, DS & Risch, SC (1984) Adrenergic-cholinergic balance and affective disorders: A review of clinical evidence and therapeutic implications. *Psychiatric Hospital, 15,* 163–71.

20. Wetterberg, L (1999) Melatonin and clinical application. *Reproduction, Nutrition, Development, 39,* 367–82.

21. Dilsaver, SC, Wetterberg, L, Blehar, MC & Rosenthal, NE (1990) Onset of winter depression earlier than generally thought? *Journal of Clinical Psychiatry, 51,* 258.

22. Blehar, MC & Rosenthal, NE (1989) Seasonal affective disorders and phototherapy. Report of a National Institute of Mental Health-sponsored workshop. *Archives of General Psychiatry, 46,* 469–74.

23. Hanh Le Quan-Bui, K, Plaisant, O, Leboyer, M, Gay, C, Kamal, L, Devynck, M-A & Meyer, P (1984) Reduced platelet serotonin in depression. *Psychiatry Research, 13*(2), 129–39.

24. Retrieved on 5/08/10 from http://www.tinnitusformula.com/infocenter/articles/treatments/trypto.aspx

25. Harrop, CE & Trower, P (2001) Why does schizophrenia develop at late adolescence? *Clinical Psychology Review, 21,* 241–65.

26. Hall, W & Degenhardt, L (2000) Cannabis use and psychosis: A review of clinical and epidemiological evidence. *Australian and New Zealand Journal of Psychiatry, 34,* 26–34. Retrieved 09/08/10 from http://www.ukcia.org/research/CannabisUseAndPsychosis.pdf

27. Shevlin, M, Murphy, J, Houston, JE & Adamson, G (2009) Childhood sexual abuse, early cannabis use and psychosis: Testing the effects of different temporal orderings based on the National Comorbidity Survey. *Psychosis, 1*(1), 19–28.

28. Read, J, Fink, P, Rudegeair, T, Felitti, V & Whitfield, C (2008) See n. 5.

29. See, for example, Moncrieff, J (2009) *A Straight Talking Introduction to Psychiatric Drugs.* Ross-on-Wye: PCCS Books.

30. Sharfstein, S (2005) Big Pharma and American psychiatry: The good, the bad and the ugly. *Psychiatr News, 40*(16), 3.

31. Shooter, M (2005) Dancing with the devil? A personal view of psychiatry's relationship with the pharmaceutical industry. *Psychiatr Bull, 29*(3), 81–3.

32. Healy, D & Thase, ME (2003) Is academic psychiatry for sale? *British Journal of Psychiatry, 182,* 388–91.

33. Mosher, LR, Gosden, R & Beder, S (2004) Drug companies and schizophrenia: Unbridled capitalism meets madness. In J Read, L Mosher & R Bentall (eds) *Models of Madness* (pp 115–30). London: Routledge.

34. Moynihan, R & Cassels, A (2005) Selling Sickness: How the world's biggest pharmaceutical companies are turning us all into patients. New York: Nation Books.

35. Mansell & Read (2009) See n. 15.

36. Read, 2008. See n. 16.

37. De Wattignar & Read, 2009. See n. 17.

38. Page 82 in Sharfstein, 2005. See n. 30.

39. Page 3 in Shooter, 2005. See n. 31.

40. Moncrieff, 2009. See n. 29.

41. Statistics from The NHS Information Centre, www.ic.nhs.uk.

42. Larkin, W & Morrison, A (eds) (2006) *Trauma and Psychosis: New directions for theory and therapy*. London: Routledge.

43. Read et al., 2008. See n. 5.

44. The Journal of the International Society for the Psychological Treatments of the Schizophrenias and other Psychoses, published by Routledge/Taylor & Francis, ISSN 1752-2439.

45. Kirsch, I, Deacon, B, Huedo-Medina, T, Scoboria, A, Moore, T & Johnson, B (2008) Initial severity and antidepressant benefits: A meta-analysis of data submitted to the Food and Drug Administration. *PLOS Medicine, 5,* 260–8.

46. Pages 5–6 in Rose, 2005. See n. 9.

47. Pages 6–7 in Rose, 2005. See n. 9.

Chapter 4

1. American Psychiatric Association (2000) *Diagnostic and Statistical Manual of Mental Disorders* (4th ed). Arlington, VA: Author.

2. Pages 92–3 in APA, 2000. See n. 1.

3. Timimi, S (2009) *A Straight Talking Introduction to Children's Mental Health Problems*. Ross-on-Wye: PCCS Books.

4. Reliability in research data is the chance of getting the same results again. Can the results be replicated or reproduced. If not the data is unreliable.

5. Page 195 in Bentall, RP (2004) Does 'schizophrenia' exist? Reliability and validity. In J Read, LR Mosher & RP Bentall (eds) *Models of Madness* (pp 43–56). London: Routledge.

6. Validity in research is when results are what they claim to be or show what they claim to show, e.g., does a diagnostic category refer to a single illness that has been demonstrated, without question, to exist?

7. Page 196 in Bentall, 2004. See n. 5.

8. Copeland JRM, Cooper, JE, Kendell, RE & Gourlay, AJ (1971) Differences in usage of diagnostic labels amongst psychiatrists in the British Isles. *Br J Psychiatry, 118,* 629–40.

9. Rosenhan, D (1975) On being sane in insane places. *Science, 179,* 250–8.

10. Slater, L (2004) *Opening Skinner's Box: Great psychological experiments of the twentieth century.* New York: Norton.

11. Herron, W et al. (1992) A comparison of 16 systems to diagnose schizophrenia. *J Clin Psychol, 48,* 711–21.

12. Page 167 in Bourdieu, P (1977) *Outline of a Theory of Practice.* Cambridge: Cambridge University Press.

Chapter 5

1. Read, J, Haslam, N, Sayce, L, & Davies, E (2006) Prejudice and schizophrenia: A review of the 'Mental illness is an illness like any other' approach. *Acta Psychiatrica Scandinavica, 114,* 303–18.

2. Page 29 in Rogers, D & Pilgrim, D (1997) The contribution of lay knowledge to the understanding and promotion of mental health. *Journal of Mental Health, 6,* 23–36.

3. Page 218 in Furnham, A & Rees, J (1988) Lay theories of schizophrenia. *International Journal of Social Psychiatry, 34*, 212–20.

4. Furnham, A & Bower, P (1992) A comparison of academic and lay theories of schizophrenia. *British Journal of Psychiatry, 161*, 201–10.

5. Page 207 in Furnham & Bower, 1992. See n. 4.

6. Page 206 in Furnham & Bower, 1992. See n. 4.

7. Page 152 in Barry, M & Greene, S (1992) Implicit models of mental disorder. *Irish Journal of Psychology, 13,* 141–60.

8. Jorm, A, Christensen, H & Griffiths, K (2005) Public beliefs about causes and risk factors for mental disorders. *Social Psychiatry & Psychiatric Epidemiology, 40*, 764–67.

9. Angermeyer, M & Dietrich, S (2006). Public beliefs about and attitudes towards people with mental illness: A review of population studies. *Acta Psychiatrica Scandinavica, 113,* 163–79.

10. Geekie, J & Read, J (2009) *Making Sense of Madness: Contesting the*

meaning of schizophrenia. London: Routledge.

11. Geekie, J, Randal, P, Lampshire, D & Read, J (in press). *Experiencing psychosis*. London: Routledge.

12. Romme, M, Escher, S, Dillon, J, Corstens, D, Morris, M (eds) (2009) *Living with Voices: 50 stories of recovery*. Ross-on-Wye: PCCS Books.

13. Bullimore, P (2010) My personal experience of psychosis. *Psychosis: Psychological, Social and Integrative Approaches, 2,* 173–7.

14. Dillon, J (2010) The tale of an ordinary little girl. *Psychosis: Psychological, Social and Integrative Approaches, 2,* 79–83.

15. Page 159 in van Dorn, R, Swanson, J, Elbogen, E & Swartz, M (2005) A comparison of stigmatizing attitudes toward persons with schizophrenia in four stakeholder groups: Perceived likelihood of violence and desire for social distance. *Psychiatry: Interpersonal and Biological Processes, 68*, 152–63.

16. Holzinger, A, Loffler, W, Muller, P, Priebe, S & Angermeyer, M (2002) Subjective illness theory and antipsychotic medication compliance by patients with schizophrenia. *Journal of Nervous & Mental Disease, 190*, 597–603.

17. Pistrang, N & Barker, C (1992) Clients' beliefs about psychological problems. *Counselling Psychology Quarterly, 5*, 325–35.

18. McCabe, R & Priebe, S (2004) Explanatory models of illness in schizophrenia: Comparison of four ethnic groups. *British Journal of Psychiatry, 185*, 25–30.

19. Read, J & Magliano, L (in press) The subjective experience and beliefs of relatives of people who experience psychosis. In J Geekie et al. (eds) *Experiencing psychosis*. London: Routledge.

20. Angermeyer, M, Klusmann, D & Walpuski, O (1988) The causes of functional psychoses as seen by patients and their relatives: II: The relatives' point of view. *European Archives of Psychiatry and Neurological Sciences, 238*, 55–61.

21. Magliano, L, De Rosa, C, Fiorillo, A, Malangone, C, Guarneri, M, Marasco, C et al. (2004) Beliefs of psychiatric nurses about schizophrenia: A comparison with patients' relatives and psychiatrists. *International Journal of Social Psychiatry, 50*, 319–30.

22. Karanci, A (1995) Caregivers of Turkish schizophrenic patients: Causal attributions, burdens and attitudes to help from the health professions. *Social Psychiatry and Psychiatric Epidemiology, 30*, 261–8.

23. Srinivasan, TN & Thara, R (2001) Beliefs about causation of schizophrenia: Do Indian families believe in supernatural causes? *Social Psychiatry and Psychiatric Epidemiology, 36*(3), 134–40.

24. Cozolino, L, Goldstein, M, Nuechterlein, W, West, K & Snyder, K (1988) The impact of education about schizophrenia on relatives varying in expressed emotion. *Schizophrenia Bulletin, 14,* 675–87.

25. McGill, C, Falloon, I, Boyd, J & Wood-Siverio, C (1983) Family educational intervention in the treatment of schizophrenia. *Hospital & Community Psychiatry, 34*, 934–8.

26. For example, Angermeyer, M & Matschinger, H (2005) Causal beliefs and attitudes to people with schizophrenia: Trend analysis based on data from two population surveys in Germany. *British Journal of Psychiatry, 186*, 331–4.

27. Read et al., 2006. See n.1.

28. Read, J, 2007. Why promoting biological ideology increases prejudice against people labelled 'schizophrenic'. *Australian Psychologist, 42*, 118–28.

29. Walker, I & Read, J (2002) The differential effectiveness of psychosocial and biogenetic causal explanations in reducing negative attitudes toward 'mental illness'. *Psychiatry: Interpersonal and Biological Processes, 65*, 313–25.

30. Page 59 in Joint Commission on Mental Illness and Health (1961) *Action for Mental Health*. New York: Basic Books.

Chapter 6

1. Read, J (2004) Poverty, ethnicity and gender. In J Read, L Mosher & R Bentall (eds) *Models of Madness* (pp 161–94). London: Routledge.

2. Kohn, M (1976) The interaction of social class and other factors in the etiology of schizophrenia. *Am J Psychiatry, 133*, 177–80.

3. Hollingshead, AB & Redlich, FC (1954) Schizophrenia and social structure. *American Journal of Psychiatry 110*, 695–701.

4. Page 177 in Kohn, 1976. See n. 2.

5. Eaton, W (1980) A formal theory of selection for schizophrenia. *Am J Sociol, 86*, 149–58.

6. Read, 2004. See n. 1.

7. Harrison G, Gunnell, D, Glazebrook, C et al. (2001) Association between schizophrenia and social inequality at birth. *Br J Psychiatry, 179,* 346–50.

8. Read, J (in press) Can poverty drive you mad? 'Schizophrenia', socio-economic status and the case for primary prevention. *New Zealand Journal of Psychology*.

9. Fortney, J, Rushton, G, Wood, S, Zhang, L, Xu, S, Dong, F & Rost, K (2007) Community-level risk factors for depression hospitalizations. *Administration and Policy in Mental Health and Mental Health Services Research, 34*, 343–52.

10. Stansfield, S, Clark, C, Rodgers, B, Caldwell, T & Power, C (2008) Childhood and adulthood socio-economic position and midlife depressive and anxiety disorders. *British Journal of Psychiatry, 192*, 152–3.

11. Wilkinson, R & Pickett, K (2009) *The Spirit Level: Why more equal societies almost always do better.* London: Allen Lane. See also the website of the Equality Trust: http://www.equalitytrust.org.uk/

12. James, O (2007) *Affluenza*. London: Vermillion.

13. Read, 2004. See n. 1.

14. Pedersen, C & Mortensen, P (2001) Urbanization and schizophrenia. *Schizophrenia Research Suppl, 41*, 65–6.

15. Read, 2004. See n. 1.

16. Read, 2004. See n. 1.

17. Read, 2004. See n. 1.

18. Janssen, I, Hanssen, M, Bak, M, Bijl, R, De Graaf, R, Vollebergh, W et al. (2003) Discrimination and delusional ideation. *British Journal of Psychiatry, 182*, 71–6.

19. Tinghog, P, Hemmingsson, T & Lundberg, I (2007) To what extent may the association between immigrant status and mental illness be explained by socioeconomic factors? *Social Psychiatry & Psychiatric Epidemiology, 42*, 990–6.

20. Read, J, Fink, P, Rudegeair, T, Felitti, V & Whitfield, C (2008) Child maltreatment and psychosis: A return to a genuinely integrated bio-psycho-social model. *Clinical Schizophrenia and Related Psychoses, 7*, 235–54.

21. Read, J, van Os, J, Morrison, A & Ross, C (2005) Childhood trauma, psychosis and schizophrenia: A literature review with theoretical and clinical implications. *Acta Psychiatrica Scandinavica, 112,* 330–50.

22. Larkin, W & Morrison, A (eds) (2006) *Trauma and Psychosis: New directions for theory and therapy*. London: Routledge.

23. Read et al., 2008. See n. 20.

24. Mullen, P, Martin, J, Anderson, J, Romans, S & Herbison, G (1993) Childhood sexual abuse and mental health in adult life. *British Journal of Psychiatry, 163*, 721–32.

25. Read, J, Agar, K, Barker-Collo, S, Davies, E & Moskowitz, A (2001) Assessing suicidality in adults: Integrating childhood trauma as a major risk factor. *Professional Psychology: Research and Practice, 32*, 367–72.

26. Read et al., 2008. See n. 20.

27. Bebbington, P, Bhugra, D, Brugha, T, Singleton, N, Farrell, M, Jenkins, R et al. (2004) Psychosis, victimization and childhood disadvantage: Evidence from the second British National Survey of Psychiatric Morbidity. *British Journal of Psychiatry, 185*, 220–6.

28. Larkin & Morrison, 2006. See n. 22.

29. Read et al., 2008. See. n. 20.

30. Larkin & Morrison, 2006. See n. 22.

31. Larkin, W & Read, J (2008) Childhood trauma and psychosis: Evidence, pathways, and implications. *Journal of Postgraduate Medicine, 54*, 284–90.

32. Read et al., 2008. See n. 20.

33. Morgan, C, Kirkbride, J, Leff, J, Craig, T, Hutchinson, G, McKenzie, K et al. (2007) Parental separation, loss and psychosis in different ethnic groups: A case-control study. *Psychological Medicine, 37*, 495–503.

34. Read, J & Gumley, A (2008) Can attachment theory help explain the relationship between childhood adversity and psychosis? *Attachment: New Directions in Psychotherapy and Relational Psychoanalysis, 2*, 1–35.

Chapter 7

1. Page 16 in Sanders, P (2006) *The Person-Centred Counselling Primer*. Ross-on-Wye: PCCS Books.

2. Masson, J (1984) *The Assault on Truth: Freud and the seduction theory*. New York: Farrar, Straus & Giroux.

3. For example, Storr, A (2001) *Freud: A very short introduction. New York: Oxford University Press.*

4. Bowlby, J (1997) *Attachment and Loss. Vol 1: Attachment* (rev 2nd ed). London: Pimlico; (1998) *Attachment and Loss. Vol 2: Separation* (new ed). London: Pimlico; (1997) *Attachment and Loss: Vol 3: Loss* (new ed). London: Pimlico.

5. Bowlby, J (1951). *Child Care and the Growth of Love*. Harmondsworth: Penguin.

6. Pages 147–55 in Cervonem D & Pervin, L (2008) *Personality: Theory and research* (10th ed). Hoboken, NJ: Wiley.

7. Fonagy, P, Gyorgy, G, Jurist, EL & Target, M (2004) *Affect Regulation, Mentalization and the Development of Self*. London: Karnac.

8. Alloy, L & Abramson, L (1979) Judgement of contingency in depressed and non-depressed students: Sadder but wiser? *Journal of Experimental Psychology: General, 108*, 441–85.

9. Haaga, D & Beck, A (1995) Perspectives on depressive realism. *Behaviour Research and Therapy, 33*, 41–8.

10. Existentialism is a philosophical approach with a very wide variety of thought, some of it contradicting other parts. Its key themes are the stress upon lived experience, freedom and the consequent task of living one's life under one's own responsibility. Philosopher Søren Kierkegaard is now regarded as the 'father of existentialism'. Wikipedia is as good a place to start as any to discover more about philosophers and schools of philosophy.

11. Phenomenology is a philosophical approach to understanding and psychology where 'truth' or 'knowledge' comes from the perceptual field of the individual, rather than an external authority. Based on work of philosopher Edmund Husserl. Again, Wikipedia is as good a place to start as any to discover more about philosophers and schools of philosophy.

Endnotes pp. 88–120

12. Carl Rogers proposed six conditions that, if present in a relationship are 'necessary and sufficient' for therapeutic change. The conditions are: (i) that the two people are in psychological contact; (ii) that one identifies themselves as the client; (iii) the other as the therapist; (iv) the therapist must be non-judgemental and warm; (v) the therapist must try to understand the client (be empathic); and (vi) the client must experience these qualities in the therapist. You can find out more about Carl Rogers and person-centred therapy in Sanders, P (2006) *The Person-Centred Counselling Primer*. Ross-on-Wye: PCCS Books.

13. Page 517 in Rogers, CR (1951) *Client-Centered Therapy: Its current practice, implications, and theory*. London: Constable. Also see n. 12.

14. For more about Carl Rogers, see Kirschenbaum, H (2007) *The Life and Work of Carl Rogers*. Ross-on-Wye: PCCS Books.

15. For research evidence, see Cooper, M, Watson, JC & Hölldampf, D (2010) *Person-Centered and Experiential Therapies Work*. Ross-on-Wye: PCCS Books.

Chapter 8

1. Klein, D, Lewinsohn, P, Seeley, R & Rohde, P (2001) A family study of major depressive disorder in a community sample of adolescents. *Archives of General Psychiatry, 58*, 13–20.

2. Rampello, L, Nicoletti, F & Nicolletti, F (1990) Dopamine and depression: Therapeutic implications. *CNS Drugs, 13,* 35–45.

3. Schatzberg, A (2002) Brain imaging in affective disorders: More questions about causes versus effects. *American Journal of Psychiatry, 159*, 1807–8.

4. Fortney, J, Rushton, G, Wood, S, Zhang, L, Xu, S, Dong, F & Rost, K (2007) Community-level risk factors for depression hospitalizations. *Administration and Policy in Mental Health and Mental Health Services Research, 34*, 343–52.

5. Albee, G (1985) The argument for primary prevention. *Journal of Primary Prevention, 5,* 213–19.

6. Davies, E & Burdett, J (2004) Preventing 'schizophrenia': Creating the conditions for saner societies. In J Read, L Mosher & R Bentall (eds) *Models of Madness* (pp 271–82). London: Routledge.

Chapter 9

1. http://www.who.int/whr/2001/en/

2. http://www.ic.nhs.uk/pubs/mentalhealth04

3. Page 1131 in Albee, G (1996) Revolutions and counter-revolutions in prevention. *American Psychologist, 51*, 1130–3.

4. Page 33 in Wilkinson, R & Pickett, K (2009) *The Spirit Level: Why more equal societies almost always do better*. London: Allen Lane.

Further Reading

The next step in understanding the causes of mental health problems is to follow your own interests. We have made suggestions under a few headings, but if you have access to the Internet, you will be able to research topics yourself.

General psychology

Richard Gross (2010) *Psychology: The science of mind and behaviour* (6th revised ed). London: Hodder Education.

'Abnormal' psychology

Paul Bennett (2006) *Abnormal and Clinical Psychology: An introductory text* (2nd ed). Buckingham: Open University Press.

Richard Bentall (2004) *Madness Explained: Psychosis and human nature.* London: Penguin.

Psychiatry

Neel Burton (2010) *Psychiatry* (2nd ed). Chichester: Wiley-Blackwell.

Critical psychology

Dennis R Fox, Isaac Prilleltensky & Stephanie Austin (2009) *Critical Psychology: An introduction* (2nd ed). London: Sage Publications.

Radical texts

Thomas Szasz (2010) *The Myth of Mental Illness* (Revised ed). New York: Harper Collins. (The original was published in 1961)

Craig Newnes, Guy Holmes & Cailzie Dunn (1999) *This is Madness: A critical look at psychiatry and the future of mental health services.* Ross-on-Wye: PCCS Books.

Subject Index

U

unconditional acceptance 121
unconscious 101
unemployment 35, 37, 50, 80, 84, 130,
        135
UNICEF 142
urbanicity 83

V

validity 62
vicarious learning 114
violence 13, 24, 26, 28, 36, 77, 85–8, 130,
        135
voluntary behaviour 111

W

women 13, 18, 22, 23, 25, 26, 29, 54, 84,
        85, 86, 87
Word War II 106, 115
World Health Organisation 55, 106, 142

Y

York Retreat 29

Name Index

Index

Index

Related reading from PCCS Books

Mental Health Madness: New perspectives for modern practice
Steven Walker (ed)
978 1 906254 44 5
(Due early 2013)

Power, Interest and Psychology: Elements of a social materialist understanding of distress
David Smail
978 1 898059 71 4
(2005)

This is Madness: A critical look at psychiatry and the future of mental health services
Craig Newnes, Guy Holmes & Cailzie Dunn (eds)
978 1 898059 25 7
(1999)

This is Madness Too: Critical perspectives on mental health services
Craig Newnes, Guy Holmes & Cailzie Dunn (eds)
978 1 898059 37 0
(2001)

Beyond Help: A consumers' guide to psychology
Susan Hansen, Alec McHoul and Mark Rapley
978 1 898059 54 7
(2003)